PRAISE FOR *FIGHT READY*

"Santino DeFranco draws on his more than twenty years of experience as an MMA fighter and coach to create a book that incorporates a cerebral sports science approach to help form a complete athlete. What does the above stammer mean? It means Santino knows what he is talking about. That his training philosophy takes into account the physical and mental aspects of training for sport."

—Forrest Griffin, UFC champion, UFC Hall of Famer, and two-time *New York Times* bestselling author

"Santino's been in my corner through every war—inside and outside the cage. He's pushed me past my limits, kept me sharp, and never let me forget who I am. Without him, I'm not the fighter—or the woman—I am today."

—Tracy Cortez, UFC women's top-ranked Flyweight fighter

"One day during a training camp, I felt fatigued and couldn't get my heart rate above 155 bpm. I kept pushing harder and harder until Coach Santino came over and told me my heart rate was a sign of overtraining, not me 'being in great shape' as I thought. That simple moment changed the camp and how I now view MMA in many ways. Coach Santino is always trying to get us to fight smarter, not just harder. I cannot recommend him and his coaching methods enough."

—The Korean Zombie, UFC Featherweight superstar and title challenger

FIGHT READY

AN MMA COACH'S GUIDE TO LOSING WEIGHT, GETTING STRONG, AND KICKING ASS

SANTINO DEFRANCO

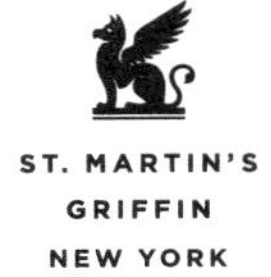

ST. MARTIN'S
GRIFFIN
NEW YORK

First published in the United States by St. Martin's Griffin, an imprint of St. Martin's Publishing Group

EU Representative: Macmillan Publishers Ireland Ltd, 1st Floor, The Liffey Trust Centre, 117–126 Sheriff Street Upper, Dublin 1, D01 YC43

www.stmartins.com

Designed by Omar Chapa

The Library of Congress Cataloging-in-Publication Data is available upon request.

ISBN 978-1-250-37800-2 (trade paperback)
ISBN 978-1-250-37801-9 (ebook)

First Edition: 2026

10 9 8 7 6 5 4 3 2 1

To Kamuela Kirk and Tracy Cortez. My need to see them reach the top of our sport led me to seek out most of the information I learned to write this book. They were my muses, my guinea pigs, and my inspiration.

Also, to my wife, Kindal, and our sons, Enzo and Lennox. They pull me out of the depths of the trenches whenever I fall too deep. They are my support system, my happiness, and my why.

The content in this book is intended solely for informational purposes and does not constitute medical advice. You should consult your doctor or healthcare professional before embarking on a new weight loss, exercise, or nutrition program and in other matters regarding your health.

CONTENTS

FOREWORD

by Henry Cejudo

I've been around a lot of coaches over the years, first in my training as a wrestler and then in my career as a mixed martial artist, and the thing I believe separates the best coaches from the rest is that first and foremost, they're teachers. I love teachers. Guys that can really break down technique in a scientific way. Santino DeFranco takes it to a whole other level. He's kind of like a professor who turns the gym into a classroom. Into a laboratory. He loves technology, sport science, and film study, and he brings them into our training camps and really digs deeply into the technical aspects of things, which is very uncommon in our sport. This book is a great illustration of that.

That's only one of the things that separates Santino from other coaches in our sport, though. Santino also knows how to work with fighters individually, according to their specific characteristics and skill sets. He's not going to work with me in the same way that he might work with a tall fighter, or with someone who doesn't have the wrestling background I have. Instead, he creates a training plan that's tailored to my specific body type and my style of fighting. And on top of that, he has the ability to push my buttons when I need it the most. So while there's a calmness to him that I appreciate, Santino also knows when he has to bring the storm. And he knows when because he knows *me*. Sometimes it's as if he knows me better than I do, which is crazy. But it speaks to the kind of guy he is. And because he knows me so well, he's always able to make adjustments.

A great example of this came during my fight against Marlon Moraes back in 2019. We were fighting for the UFC bantamweight title, and I was fighting at a bit of a disadvantage because I had sprained my ankle pretty badly in training a few days before. It was a rough start in round one.

After the first round, Santino made an adjustment. He said, "This is like the Demetrious round one all over again. You're in kicking range. You need to box your way in and meet him in the middle," which really swung the momentum in my direction. But then, I injured my left shoulder. I was basically fighting with one arm and one leg and, as a result, Moraes was really taking the fight to me.

I'll never forget this. I came to the corner after round two and Santino said, "Hey, listen, man, forget the game plan. You just gotta go in there and fight him. The shoulder doesn't matter. You have to stay in his face." He knew my ankle was in bad shape (I was out of training for like three months after this fight because of it) and that my only real chance to beat Moraes and claim the belt was to make it an old-fashioned street fight. Call it Mexican style. Warrior style. Whatever. I just had to go out there and eat. Santino knew it and so did I. So that's what I did. I took the fight to Moraes and stopped him in the third. TKO. And with that win I became only the fourth UFC fighter ever to hold belts in two weight classes simultaneously. And really, I owe a lot of that win to Santino. Sometimes as a fighter you need that push from a coach that is just different. For the guy to have the courage in those critical moments not to tell you what you want to hear but instead what you *need* to hear. That night he knew exactly what I needed.

Santino always says that it's important for fighters to be delusional, to have a belief in oneself that is actually a little bit unrealistic so that we can push ourselves beyond our perceived limits. That was something I felt back when I was wrestling, but if I'm being honest I never really had it in mixed martial arts until I met Santino. He just has an innate ability to make you believe that you can accomplish anything, no matter what. And we proved it that night.

I'm no psychologist, but I think a lot of that comes from Santino's own experience as a fighter. The brain aneurysm that he had, which forced him to stop fighting, also stopped him from reaching greatness, but it didn't stop him from winning. What it also did was put a big old chip on his shoulder. And he's been able to really pay that forward with a lot of us, particularly with the belief that he instills in us. He can motivate while he's teaching you things and showing you what to do and making you understand everything. And he's able to cut through all the noise and keep you focused on the objective, which is winning. Santino is a winner, man.

I've reached the highest level in sports. The cream of the crop. And what I've noticed along the way is that sometimes the reason why people don't succeed is because they don't have the right engineers. When you have a proper engineer who understands biomechanics, who understands the importance of recovery, nutrition, sleep—all of that—it changes the game. This became clear to me as soon as Santino entered our camp for my second fight against Demetrious Johnson. I mean, talk about going from A to Z right away. He came into the camp and immediately started making adjustments. He could tell that I had been overtraining (which I was known to do, often to my great detriment) and dialed things way back. We studied film, and we spent hours every week watching Johnson's previous fights so I could learn and prepare to counteract his tendencies. And then there was the soothing comfort of knowing that I finally had a coach who was ready to launch me and give me the kind of confidence you can only feel when you're fully prepared. I recognized right away that he was a high-level engineer. That he was a mechanic for Ferraris and Lamborghinis, which is what I've always been. I've always been a Ferrari. But I was working with Honda mechanics before I met Santino. It's not until you really get a Ferrari or a Lamborghini mechanic that you realize the difference. And with Santino in my corner I accomplished something few believed I could, especially after the way my first fight with Johnson ended. This time I ended his incredible streak of eleven consecutive title defenses and claimed the UFC Flyweight title. It was Johnson's first loss in more than six years.

What makes Santino really special, I think, is that he's smart enough to know that he doesn't know everything. So he finds people who do. He understands his role, and he understands what isn't his role. Santino focused on the MMA side of camp, but he communicated with the UFC performance institute coaches and dieticians so that everyone was always on the same page. Then, when it came to the strength and conditioning part of training, he listened. We worked with an outside S and C group and tracked every biometric there was, and then he held me accountable to what all of the data pointed to. Besides all of the numbers, he knew that I needed to feel good while I was training. So he'd actually ask me how I was feeling and what changes I thought were needed. He knew that I had a tendency to overtrain to the point that, once or twice, I had to be carried out of the gym on a stretcher due to back spasms, and he wasn't having any of that. He wanted me to get to the sparring phase of training feeling good. Feeling 100 percent, so that when fight night came, I was at my best. We both knew that the best way to achieve that was for me to feel like he and I were truly in sync. That we were equal partners who were in it together. Because that second fight against Demetrious Johnson wasn't only the biggest fight of my career, it was the biggest fight of his career, too. We both had a lot on the line.

My Olympic coach was one of a kind, and he helped me achieve my dream of winning an Olympic gold medal. The youngest American wrestler ever to take the gold. But I think what Santino taught me is that there are different paths to success. You don't always need a drill sergeant. You don't always need somebody who's gonna be jumping down your throat, or kicking you in the ass, because it's different when you get older. That kind of approach will burn you out. I think what Santino brings to the table is a lot of new age coaching. He's always learning, always adjusting, always trying to find that competitive edge. And in a sport where the margin for error is basically zero, that's a really fresh perspective. Santino has a real gift for teaching in a way that makes his fighters buy-in fully. He makes disciples out of us. Other coaches can lead you to water, but Santino makes you want to drink it. He trusts me to understand that it's ultimately up to me. It's my career. How do I want my book to be written?

Would Michael Jordan have achieved what he did without Phil Jackson? Would Phil Jackson have achieved what he did without Michael Jordan and, later, Kobe Bryant? I doubt it. Talent can only take an athlete or coach so far. To succeed at the highest level, it takes that perfect synergy. It takes mutual trust and respect. And then, once you find that coach, it's all different. Everything changes. It's like the whole world slows down.

I hope that's what this book does for you, so that you, too, can perform at your very best when your very best is needed. This book is a perfect distillation of everything Santino DeFranco is and what he believes, and I can't wait to see what you can accomplish with Santino in your corner. You're the Ferrari now.

—Henry Cejudo, Olympic Gold Medalist and two-division UFC champion

FIGHT READY

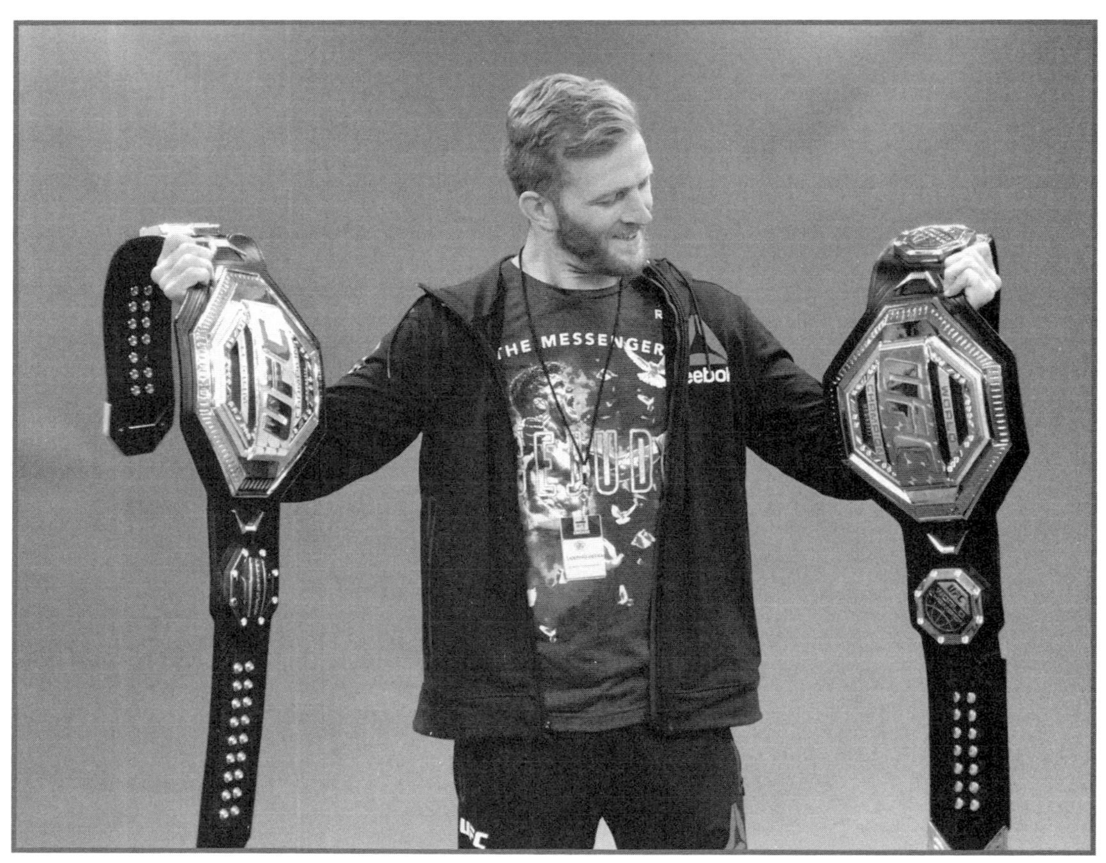

Here I am sporting both belts after Henry Cejudo won his second weight division UFC championship.

Seigher Brown

INTRODUCTION

What It Means to Be Fight Ready

To be "fight ready" is to exist in a state of optimal physical and mental preparedness that enables a fighter to execute and perform at a peak level at the moment when his or her best is required. As a trainer of elite mixed martial artists who knows firsthand how slim the margin for error is, my mission is to build fighters up, through a combination of diet, nutrition, conditioning, strength, skills, rest, and mental fortitude, to achieve a fight ready state at the moment of the fight, so they can go out and dominate their opponent and the moment.

Achieving your athletic goal is going to take a combination of purpose, strength and conditioning, diet and nutrition, and well-organized training plans. I am going to help you with all of those, and I am going to help you to become fight ready.

PART ONE

What's Your Fight?

What are you fighting for? Why are you here? We all have goals. Some of us want to look good in a summer bikini or a wedding dress. Or maybe we want to lose twenty pounds or place in the local 5K race or CrossFit competition. Maybe we're a weekend warrior or even a pro or semipro athlete. Maybe we're not an athlete at all, but instead trying to start a business? Goals are goals regardless, and achieving those goals in a sport is similar to achieving goals in business or as a creative. But achieving those goals sometimes seems so difficult that we don't even start, or we don't know how to. And if we do start, we often find ourselves lost along the way. Perhaps we know where we want to go, but for one reason or another we can't seem to get to the finish line.

That's why I'm here. I've helped fighters like Henry Cejudo, Kelvin Gastelum, Korean Zombie, and Tracy Cortez to their goal of competing at the highest level of their sport, and I can guide you to your goals as well. But before I send you off on your journey, you'll first need to be prepared because, otherwise, you'd fail faster than you did the last time you tried to give up soda for a month. If I just sent you into section two or three of this book and said eat this and lift that, there's no question that you'd fail. You wouldn't be prepared for what you were about to go through—not even remotely—and it would be entirely my fault for sending you into a fight unprepared. There's so much more to losing weight than counting calories, and there's a lot more to getting strong

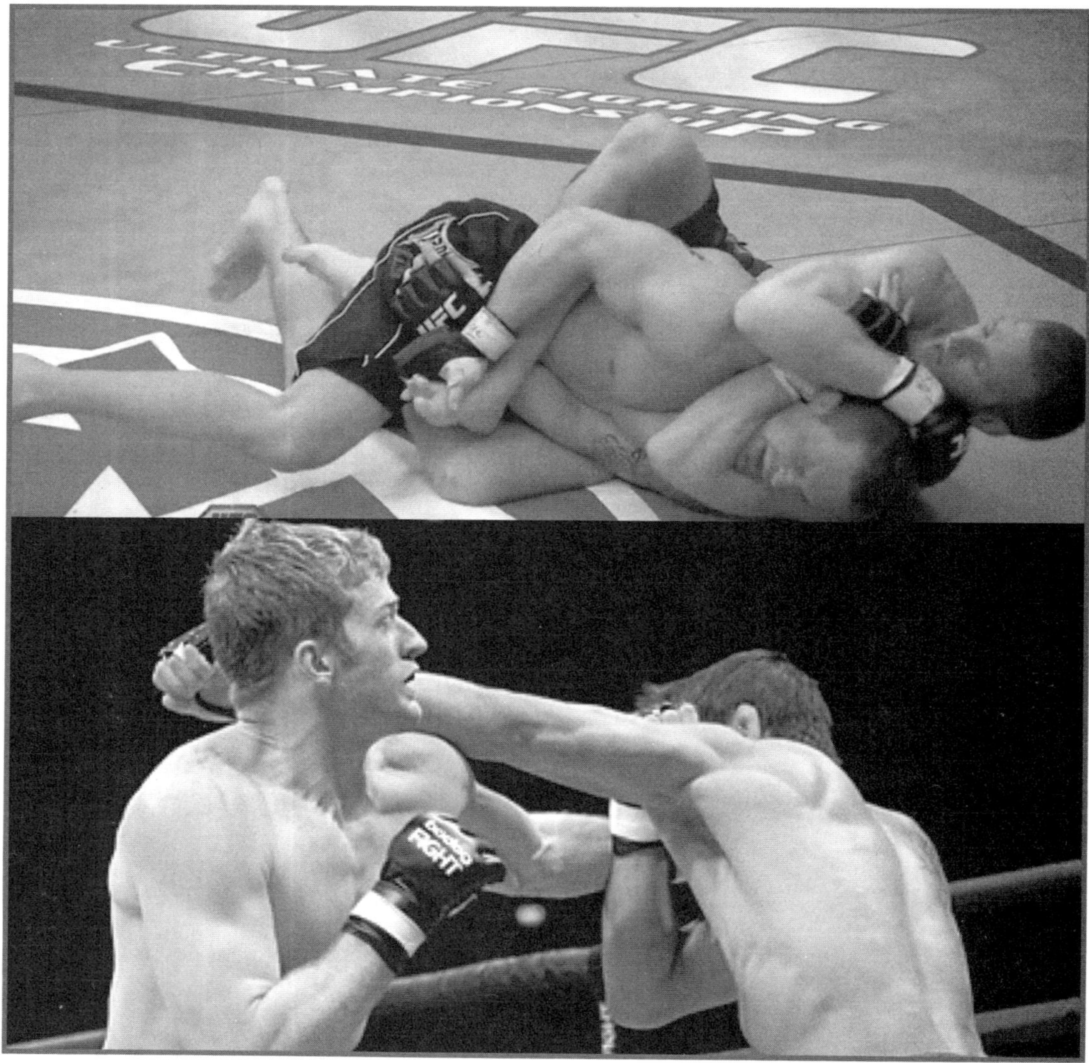

Before being diagnosed with a brain aneurysm, I was a promising fighter myself with a record of 11–2.

UFC.com (top)/Keith Mills (bottom)

than just lifting heavy things. Success requires a planned course of action, and rarely is it one-dimensional. You're going to need a holistic approach to actualize your goal—whether that goal is a sport or a business, or anything in between. If it were easy, then you wouldn't need me or this book.

First, you need to understand a few things. As kids, we all learned the saying KISS, which besides being a kick-ass glam rock band is an acronym for Keep It Simple, Stupid. That axiom remains true to this day. The most productive you'll ever be is when you're keeping it simple. Overcomplicating things is what snake oil salesmen do when they're trying to pull the wool over your eyes. Or maybe they're just misinformed? I don't know. But one of my all-time favorite quotes is from historian Daniel Boorstin, who said that "the greatest enemy of knowledge is not ignorance, it is the illusion of knowledge." There's a lot of truth in that, and the diet and fitness industries are full of supposed experts who think they know what they're doing, but don't. And as well-intentioned as some of them might be, they're leading people astray. If you are trying to gain knowledge on health, nutrition, business—anything!—by scrolling social media or by picking up the new fad diet book or exercise plan, you're going to have to sift through the dregs of nonsense and misinformation and conflicting studies to try to make sense of the best approach.

I began my own MMA journey while the sport was still in its formative years, and throughout my own experiences as a fighter, and then as I climbed my way up the coaching ladder, I've seen a near insurmountable wave of "coaches" and "experts" trying to sell their version of nutrition, strength programs, fighting systems, mental training, and every other "secret" weapon to success. These so-called "experts" sell their services, latch on to fighters, and suck out the time and money and energy of fighters and anyone attached to them who they can squeeze out a profit or social media likes from. The barrier to entry is so low in the orbit of athletics that anyone can claim to be a nutritionist or strength coach. Anyone is an expert if they can plead their case well enough. I've been pushing these people away from my own fighters for years, and I've been debunking the latest trends and fads for years now, and I'm here to help you do the same. Not only do I want to help educate you on what I've used to find success with my own fighters, but I also want to educate you on how you can discern between useful, good information and the blatantly bad information meant to make someone a quick buck. But there's more to success than just learning good technical information; you need to understand the process of that information, and how to use the information.

While the technical aspects of achieving your health and fitness goals (the specifics of diet and exercise) are critical, the tactical components (getting enough sleep, mindset, preparation, dealing with adversity) are just as important. If you don't have the tactical knowledge to handle roadblocks, you're likely going to become frustrated and quit. I already know this, so why would I allow you to start your camp knowing that you will fail? I won't. When you're out there running and lifting and dieting as scheduled but still not losing weight, we have to look at your sleep patterns, stress levels, the timing of your workouts, and so much more to devise a multifaceted plan that can achieve the desired results.

Success begins with movement, putting one foot in front of the other. Success begins when you start to move forward. That's how you gather momentum. And once you can see the light at the end of the tunnel, when you glimpse the finish line, it becomes a lot easier to push hard and through to the end. But it's in the middle distance where the bulk of success takes place. If the start of the marathon is the first three miles and the end is the same, you win or lose the race in the twenty miles in between. Those are the hardest miles. Those are the miles we're going to help you with in part one of this book.

1

BE DELUSIONAL

The best, most successful people I know, both fighters and high achievers in other fields, are all a bit delusional. They all have an innate drive to be the best they can be and believe they can and will succeed in whatever task they undertake, regardless of the obstacle or opponent. That kind of radical self-belief is powerful, and it's one of the reasons why, as George Bernard Shaw famously quipped, "all progress depends upon the unreasonable man." Only unreasonable men set out to accomplish unreasonable things, and things that have yet to be done are, to "reasonable men," inherently unreasonable.

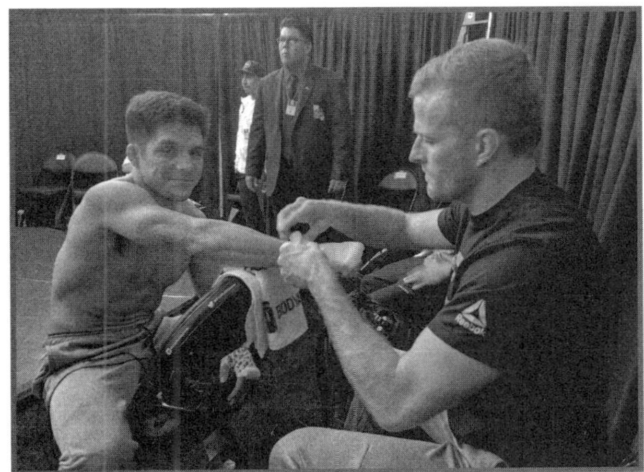

The oddsmakers didn't give Henry a shot to beat Demetrious Johnson, but he believed in his ability to win, and that's all that mattered.

Seigher Brown

In society, we often encounter delusional people who exude extreme self-confidence, and we call them crazy. The odds of being successful, let alone the best in the world, are slim. Most of us are average at best. There's a bell curve for a reason, and the law of averages tells us that. I mean, there's a law that says you won't be very successful in relation to your peers! Yet, it turns out that being somewhat delusional is a common trait among the most successful people. Ever hear of Kanye West? He's a musical genius, and an absolute madman—convinced he's the most important man in history. This group of delusional people, whether a fighter or high achiever in a different field, possess an innate drive to excel and a radical belief in their capabilities, regardless of the statistical improbability of their aspirations. This type of radical self-belief, bordering on delusion, is incredibly powerful and often propels individuals toward great achievements.

Parents, teachers, and PSAs tell kids they can be anything. They can do anything. They can achieve anything. They say to work hard, and success follows. And they're wrong. You're not special. I'm not special. He's not special. Logic tells us that. And even though we're not special, we must believe we're special. We may not all be able to become the president of the United States—only forty-five people have ever done that—but we have to believe we can become the president of the United States to reach our personal ceiling. What do they say? "Reach for the stars, and you might just land on the moon"? Even if our goal is above our ceiling, we have to crack the roof. It's our duty as sound humans to reach our individual ceilings in whatever endeavor we choose. Otherwise, we're leaving talent to waste. We must reach our ceiling!

As children, we're encouraged to be dreamers. Our parents encourage us to dream of being doctors, astronauts, or painters, but as high school and college begin, they say, "ditch the band," "ditch the art," "ditch the sports." We're supposed to temper our expectations because statistically, most of us will never become the next LeBron James or Bill Gates. And the truth is we probably won't achieve that level of success. We can only reach as high as our personal limits allow—our own personal ceiling—which, for the vast majority, is far below the heights of extraordinary achievement. Yet, it is this very delusion about our limitless potential that drives us to pursue our goals with fervor and, occasionally, achieve the seemingly impossible. We cannot accept our place on the bell curve.

Consider the story of former UFC Featherweight and lightweight champion Conor McGregor. McGregor's life was transformed after he read *The Secret*, a book about manifesting one's desires into reality. He embraced this idea wholeheartedly, despite everyone around him dismissing his ambitions as foolish. They were right, of course; he was being unreasonable—yet, McGregor harnessed the power of his own delusion to achieve something unprecedented: he became the UFC champion in two weight classes simultaneously.

And when I was saying I want to become number one of the world and I was seven, eight years old, most of the people were laughing to me. Because, it seemed like I have one percent of chances to do that. And I've done it.

—Novak Djokovic, tennis champion

McGregor believed in what others thought was impossible, and that's what helped him push forward toward success. Delusion can only get you so far without dedication, discipline, sacrifice, and endurance, which we'll talk about more in later chapters—but it's the delusion that picked him up after losses. The delusion pushed him forward through the depression and self-doubt. The delusion is the thread that carried him from one roadblock to the next. The delusion kept him failing forward as opposed to failing and quitting.

This might seem ludicrous to someone on the outside, but anyone who aspires toward greatness in any field must harbor a bit of a messiah complex—believing oneself to be "the one" even when everyone else views them as insane.

In reality, this belief is indeed a form of insanity, until, of course, you reach your goal and prove your vision was clear all along. The stark reality about human potential and achievement is much bleaker than we like to admit because only morons and the mentally insane believe they're the greatest in the world until they are. Only by nurturing this delusion can we push ourselves to fully realize our capabilities, whether in sports, business, or any other field. And while most who embrace this mindset may still fall short, they achieve far more than those who never dare to dream big.

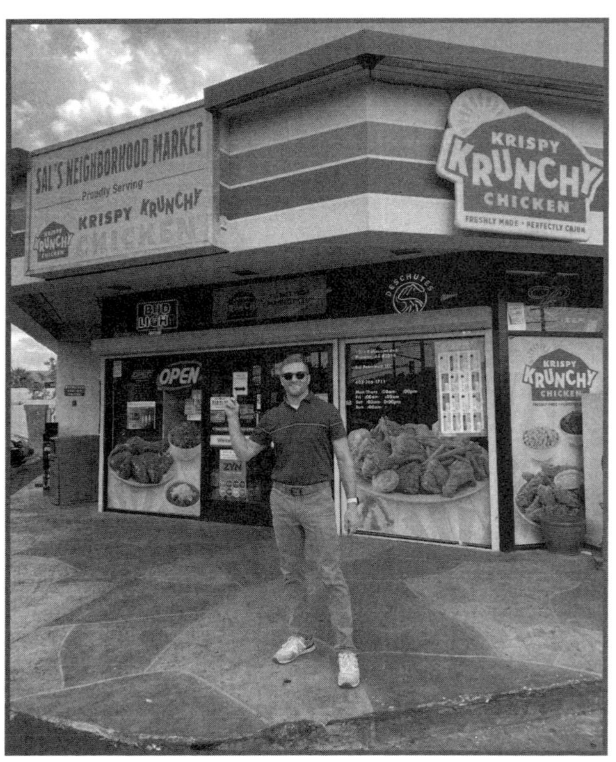

I bought a Shell-branded gas station during the pandemic, and figured it out along the way. *Seigher Brown*

TYPES OF DELUSIONS

In 2021, I bought a gas station. Covid had decimated the gym industry the previous year, and the uncertainty of the future shook my comfort level. I realized that if gyms went down for good, I'd be out of a job. And I didn't really have any other job skills. "MMA fighter and coach" on a resume doesn't exactly open the doors to a six-figure salary. I'd have to start over in a new field for much less money than I was making in MMA. It occurred to me that I didn't have control of my future or finances. The gym industry had total control over me, and I don't like being out of control.

I'd spent the previous few years

saving money and investing in the stock market, and between my savings and my wife's 401(k) that we could take a loan from, I knew I could be approved for an SBA (small business association) loan. I scoured business listings for months. Every single listing posted for six months passed through my phone or computer. I wanted something that had the right balance of cost, cash flow, and time management. Gas stations seemed to have the right blend I was looking for. But what did I know about gas stations?

Nothing. I knew nothing about gas stations. I figured if a bunch of other people could do it, I could too. Years ago, a friend, Curt Howard, a nurse at the local hospital, was in the middle of buying and renovating a house to flip. He wasn't a tradesman before. He didn't work construction for his father in high school. So, when he was telling me about changing the electrical box, replumbing the shower, and laying a slab to add an addition, I asked, "How do you know how to do all of this?" He replied, "I don't. I just YouTube it. Look, if you knew the average electrician or plumber, you'd know they aren't a bunch of geniuses. If they can do this stuff, you and I can figure it out too." That is some of the best advice I've ever received. If they can do it, I can figure it out too. It's kind of my superpower—I'm never afraid of starting something. I figure I'll learn along the way. And it's also part of the reason I don't overly plan before undertaking huge tasks (like buying a gas station)—I assume I'll figure it all out. I will just succeed. I know that. The gas station had a whole lot more "figuring out" than I thought.

The SBA loan process was painful. Home loans pale in comparison to an SBA loan. Of course, we had to supply them with all our finances (bank statements, credit checks, work history), but then they placed a lien on our home—we couldn't sell it or refinance it until the business loan was paid off. Then the bank required more down payment than we originally were told—the loan officer just assumed we'd know this. As the closing date neared, the landlord (owner of the actual building) said my net worth wasn't enough for him to rent to me (they wanted a ten-million-dollar net worth and liquid assets of two million), which I didn't have. So I had to negotiate a sublease with the seller. Then there were permits: health permits, retail permits, liquor, tobacco, environmental, state, city. They never ended. I had to apply for numerous lines of credit with various vendors and suppliers—my credit score went from 820 to 730 in weeks. The day after we closed on the station, I was told the AC had to be replaced immediately. The kitchen was supposed to be "almost ready" to use. Five months and $48,000 later, it was open. This is a fractional list of the roadblocks I encountered while purchasing the station.

I'm a few years in now, and I love owning the station. It was a great investment. But if I had any damn clue how much work and stress and chaos would go into purchasing the station—I'd have bailed. If I had looked up and seen the papers, permits, and dollar signs in front of my face with no end in sight, with no idea if it would be successful or an absolute wreck, I would have said no a million times.

If I had any clue, I'd have gone another route. But I didn't. I thought every roadblock was the last. I told my wife that every permit was the last, that every fee was the last—either to placate her fears or my own.

You have to have some sort of idea of what you want (your delusional goal), but then just keep looking down at your feet: one foot in front of the other. And when you want to look up and see how far you've gone and how far you have to go, don't. Just pay the permits.

Delusions help us dream big. They keep the youthful naivety needed to daydream of greatness. They are our dreams of owning our own business someday. But we need a lot of different delusions. Just like short-term and long-term goals, we need short-term and long-term delusions. We need delusions to help us during setbacks. We need delusions to help us stay positive when we lose and people are better than us. We need delusions to shield us from reality: The bell curve is reality. The bell curve is our enemy. It's as if we are young again, and our mom peeks in our bedroom—we cover our heads with the blanket because, remember, if we can't see them, they can't see us.

These long-term delusions are the delusions of grandeur—the McGregor "I'm going to be the best in the world" delusions. Delusions of grandeur are just part of the delusional process, though. The grandeur is the long-term goal. The world championship. The Super Bowl. The delusions of grandeur keep us looking so far into the future we don't realize the hardship right in front of us. The long-term is far off, though, and progress is made in the middle of the race. It's easy to start, and it's easy to finish.

From the start of the race to the first three miles or so, you are fresh. Fatigue isn't a factor. Your muscles are loose and fluid. Glycogen stores are high. All is well. And by the last three miles, the end is in sight. The finish line is near. It's easy to push when you see your end goal. But the middle—oh, the middle! This is where the battle is won and lost. This is when you start to hurt and slow down. How fast am I running? Can I keep this pace? Everything hurts. Injuries occur. If you look up and see there's no end in sight, panic can set in. Uncertainty can set in. The reality of the magnitude of the race sets in. Don't look up. Look down at your feet. One foot in front of the other (short-term delusions). Long-term delusions—dreaming of the finish line—are good; they are the end goal. Short-term delusions are good; they keep us looking down at our feet. They keep us from looking up during the middle of the race and realizing how lost we are. How little we've gone. How far we have to go. The short-term delusions keep us from looking up at what success actually takes: a lot of hard, grueling work for years more than what we think. They keep us from quitting when "the going gets tough."

We now know what the long-term delusions are. So what are short-term delusions, and how do we use them to our benefit?

Short-term delusions keep us motivated. They keep hope in us, one rep after another. Those delusions prevent us from accepting that the people we're training with are actually better than us. Don't accept that people are better than you.

One thought process I always had while training was the "this next rep is the one" mentality. If I was wrestling with someone who was clearly better than me, I'd get taken down (and be unable to take him down). "Alright, he got me. I'll get him this next time." But then he takes me down again and again. Five times. Six. Ten. "I'll try my double leg." Nope. Taken down. "I'll switch from my double leg to a single leg." Nope. Taken down. "He's getting tired. This next one's mine." Nope. Taken down. "Statistics alone say he won't get me 20–0." Nope. Taken down. "I'll try this." Nope. Taken down. "I'll try that." Nope, taken down. I'd keep thinking that the very next time would have to be THE time. I couldn't allow my mind to say, "He's better than me. I can't win." That mentality is death. Believing in success is paramount because as I lost one takedown after the next, I got better. Each failed attempt was a learning experience. I just kept failing forward until, one day, I actually did get the takedown. But we need to justify our losses with anything but, "He's better than me. I can't win." If we have a losing mentality, we'll lose. But if we keep delusional optimism, we'll fail forward until we find success. Success is always just one more failed rep away.

Whether you think you can, or whether you think you can't, you're right.

—Henry Ford

So, long-term delusions are the goal, and short-term delusions prevent us from looking up at the middle. But there's something else we need to account for: failures and setbacks.

We want to be blind to setbacks. We need to be delusional about our losses; otherwise, reality sets in. The bell curve rears its ugly, rooted-in-reality head, and we realize we're not exceptional. We've all heard the story of Michael Jordan not making his freshman basketball team. We've heard of Tom Brady being drafted in the sixth round. Brady famously told New England Patriots owner Robert Kraft, "I'm the best decision this organization has ever made," when meeting him for the first time (according to Kraft's retelling). "How insane is this random fourth-rate quarterback?" Kraft must have thought! One of the best boxing middleweights, Bernard Hopkins, lost his first professional fight to Clinton Mitchell, who was 0–1 at the time. Former UFC Featherweight and lightweight champion Conor McGregor lost his third professional fight to Artemij Sitenkov, an unknown fighter with a record of 5–4 when they fought. With each of these examples, how could any of them believe they were destined for greatness? Hopkins couldn't beat an 0–1 fighter, but he expects to be middleweight champion of the world? Floyd Mayweather was 50–0. Now that's a world champion! How could a guy who went sixth round in the NFL draft expect to be a starter in the league, let alone the GOAT? We need delusions for setbacks. We need to still believe we are the best even though we lost. But the logic doesn't add up. Certain losses make it look like we belong in the middle of the bell curve. We're just another competitor. We need an excuse. Not an empty excuse without change, but an excuse.

Just like we don't want to say, "He's better than me. I can't win," we also don't want to say, "He was better than me; that's why I lost." Maybe later in the career, but not early. That's a bad mindset. We want to be logical about our excuses too.

We didn't lose the race because "he's faster than me." That's not something we can control. If we say that, there's nothing we can do, and we may as well quit. We didn't lose the basketball game because "they were just better." We lost the basketball game because "we just missed too many threes. If we had just made a couple more threes, we'd have won."

"I only lost the fight because he was stronger, or my cardio wasn't as good as it should have been. My weight cut was off. Otherwise, I would have won!" I can improve my cardio. I can get stronger. I can get better. But I can't handle losing. Be a sore loser—it's better in the long run, even if people don't like to hear it.

WE NEED TO REFRAME THE NARRATIVE

All of those *are* "excuses," but they're *real* excuses. Those types of excuses give us areas of focus after each game, fight, or race to improve upon. We need to reframe why we lost and compartmentalize them into "reasons why I lost," as those are specific things we can correct. The moment we start to say, "I lost because she was better than me" is the moment we allow reality to settle us right into the bell curve. The thought of losing to a random person in anything just leads us to believe that we can't make it to that GOAT status. And even if we can't be the GOAT, remember, we all have to believe we can be. "I only lost because my cardio wasn't as good as his" may or may not be true, but it gives us something to strive for (better cardio) in our next fight. We always have to be improving. That's a given. Whether cardio, technique, or weight training—those areas always have to be trending up and to the right. We can't skimp on technical attributes. But we can't allow the thought of "someone is better than me" to take stake in our minds.

> *To be an overachiever you have to be an over-believer.*
>
> *—Dabo Swinney, Clemson football coach*

We know that the exception to the rule doesn't negate the rule. Just because people have jumped out of an airplane and their chute didn't open and they lived doesn't mean you can jump out of an airplane and expect to walk away. That's why we see successful people. Rich people. Strong people. But we say, "I can't do that" or "they can only do that because they're talented or athletic or whatever." But you must become the exception to the rule—or at least fight like hell to be.

If delusion motivates us to sign up for the 100-mile race, arrogance is what makes us think we can win.

We call them arrogant. We think they believe they're better than us, and we find that brash arrogance distasteful, even when it's expressed as strong confidence. How dare someone think they're better than me at something? Even when others genuinely surpass us in abilities or achievements, we don't want them thinking or saying they are better. We are a jealous species, craving equality especially when we witness the good-looking, wealthy, or athletically gifted succeed—unless, of course, we find ourselves in their shoes, at the top of the podium or cashing the big checks. Then, as others shout "Unfair," we claim meritocracy. We love to win, and we love to make excuses when we lose.

Confidence is what comes after success. Arrogance is what you have before you've achieved it. And you have to be arrogant to believe that you will write a *New York Times* bestseller. That you will create a billion-dollar unicorn company. That you will be world champion. But you need that too, especially when it comes down to fighting or any physical feat.

I used to train Efraín Escudero. When I met him, he was eighteen years old. full of arrogance and swagger and all the piss and vinegar you could imagine. But he was also charismatic and good-looking. He was a poor kid from Yuma. He wrestled at a junior college in Tucson, Arizona, where he placed eighth in the nation—claiming him All-American honors. He compiled an 8–0 cage record before joining and winning season 8 of the reality TV show *The Ultimate Fighter*. Escudero won his first two professional fights postshow due to his exceptional natural talent and an unwavering belief in his invincibility. He wasn't the most technically skilled fighter; his approach was more about raw power and aggression. He didn't believe he could lose. He believed he was too good to lose, and so he just didn't. He beat people who were "supposed" to dismantle him. The brash cockiness kept his hand raised until, eventually, his career took a downturn after he experienced his first major defeat against a more technically skilled and conditioned opponent, Evan Dunham, who bested him with an arm bar submission. This loss shattered his self-perception of invincibility. Knowing now that he could lose, that he could get tired and be caught, Escudero changed his fighting style. He began fighting not to lose rather than fighting to win, adjusting his pace to maintain his cardio and health rather than striving for victory. This shift highlights how even one defeat can profoundly affect an athlete's confidence and approach to their sport.

SOMEBODY HAS TO BE GREAT . . . IT MAY AS WELL BE YOU

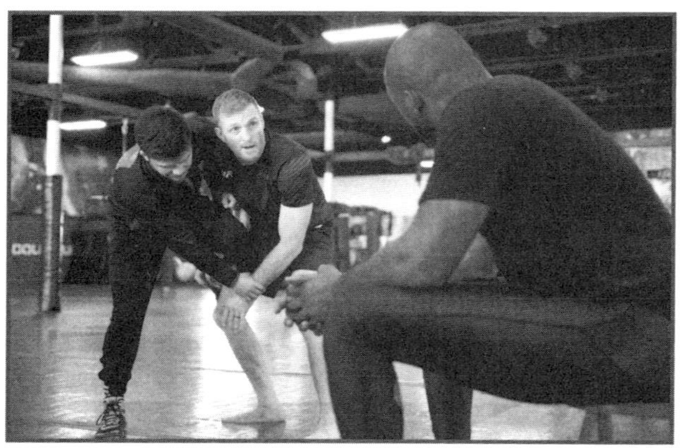

If someone has to be great, it may as well be you. Here I am with Jon Jones and Henry Cejudo, two of MMA's greatest fighters to ever do it. *Seigher Brown*

Though we may disparage arrogance and delusion in our everyday encounters, these traits are often the hallmarks of those who transcend ordinary bounds to achieve extraordinary success. The path to greatness is paved with unreasonable beliefs and, quite often, a stubborn refusal to acknowledge limits. Delusion will get you to sign up for the race. Arrogance will get you to the finish line. But if you want to be on the podium, you need dedication, discipline, sacrifice, and endurance.

2

SLEEP IS A SUPER DRUG

It's been nearly thirty years since Nas famously rapped "I never sleep, cuz sleep is the cousin of death." But while that's a heck of a line, poor sleep habits might spell a fighter's actual (or figurative) death in the cage. Long gone are the days of "there's no rest for the wicked." Bragging about pulling all-nighters (or even sleeping just a few hours) and then going to work or to football practice or to school is as cool as talking about how many beers you shotgunned at the frat party last night. These days, I'm not high-fiving you. I'm rolling my eyes and walking the other direction. I get it. And we've all done it. But poor sleep ruins lives. Athletically, but also . . . kind of in every aspect of life. We're not in high school or college anymore, and burning the candle at both ends just isn't cool like it used to be. Plan your day like an adult. Sleep like an adult. Perform like a champion. It's time to scare you straight into bed. Sleep is not a passive activity. The brain isn't hibernating and the body isn't lifeless. Think of sleep as the cocoon. From the outside, it may appear dormant, but a magnificent amount of life and energy is occurring—we just don't see it until the butterfly breaks out.

Every member of the animal kingdom requires basic needs for life: food, water, oxygen, shelter, and sleep. How can we expect to optimize in any area if we can't even get all those basic needs down? If we're operating in a food deficit or water deficit, we're not going to perform. Same goes for sleep. But if we zoom in even further, we spend nearly one third of our lives asleep! Sleep is *that* important. But why? And why are we ignoring one third of our lives and acting like it doesn't exist, or at the very best, that it's something passive that just occurs—like software running in the background of our computer that we never really realize is there?

BEYOND ATHLETICS

Having one bad night of sleep (or even a few days of bad sleep), which would not be considered an "acute sleep disorder," won't kill you, even if it does wreak havoc on your system in the short term, but chronic sleep disorders (less than seven hours of sleep a night for one to three months) certainly may. Sleep—or lack thereof—has been linked to numerous physiological diseases: hypertension, coronary artery disease, obesity, and diabetes, among others. In addition to physical ailments, chronic lack of sleep has also been linked to "negative mood and mood regulation, psychosis, anxiety, suicidal behavior, and the risk for depression." Sleep isn't just needed to wake up feeling fresh for that math test in tenth grade. It's everything. It really is the super drug. And if quality sleep will turn you into Superman, consider lack of sleep, or poor sleep, Lex Luthor with a handful of kryptonite.

But you're not here for the let's-be-healthy-over-thirty speech, although this book is really about lifestyle changes and life habits—you're here for the how will better sleep help me lose weight/win competitions/be more athletic speech—I have to admit, though, my hypocrisy will rear its head later when I go over the weight cutting and how to try to get as close to death as possible—but I digress.

WHY WE SLEEP

The "too long; didn't read" version is . . . we think we're on the right track to knowing, but scientists aren't all in agreement. Conceivably, most of what occurs during sleep could occur during a state of wakefulness. We definitely have a lot of ideas, and different phases of sleep are attributed to different physiological processes. One theory is that during sleep our brains filter out toxins and by-products of the day's workload (adenosine). Similar to how the anaerobic muscle by-product is lactic acid and buffering that acid is important to recovery and continued use, the brain needs a recovery process too. Then the memory consolidation and learning processes that occur in phase two through the rise of sleep spindles (different types of brain waves), then physiological rebuilding of tissue that occurs in phase three. But REM (rapid-eye movement) sleep? The subject of controversy and mystique for millennia. The best we can do is, well . . . the best we can do. But the actual knowledge of the subject of sleep is more theory and guesswork than hard evidence that the medical community as a whole agrees on.

A BRIEF HISTORY

For as long as creatures have been sleeping, there has been a surprising lack of understanding of the bodily state. You'd think that for how ubiquitous sleep is, we'd know a bit more about it. And although the curiosity has been there, the knowledge and study has been limited. Early humans acknowledged sleep, especially REM sleep, but focused more on dreams and their meanings—attributing the phenomena to demons and angering or pleasing the gods. Using dreams as visions to send warning signs to those who had them, as opposed to attaching them to physiologically normal occurrences of the body's daily cycle of life.

In about 400 BC, scholars linked a drop in body temperature to sleep.

Later, Aristotle, in approximately 350 BC, acknowledged a connection between human fevers and lethargy, linking the immune system and digestive system to sleep. He (incorrectly) postulated that the drop in heart rate caused a person to sleep, though he was correct that the heart rate does decrease during sleep, and other sleep components were identified—drop in temperature, changes in digestive processes, paralysis during REM sleep. But so many pieces of the sleep puzzle were missing, or put into the wrong order of operations.

It wasn't until thousands of years later that scientists began to have a clearer understanding of sleep. In 1729, Jean Jacques d'Ortuous de Mairan discovered the circadian rhythm while studying plants, and it wasn't until almost two hundred years after that, in the early 1900s, that real sleep study took off within the medical and scientific community. Which isn't really surprising seeing as how little most people even know about sleep, or its importance today in 2025. Out of sight, out of mind is so prominent in this situation.

This isn't a textbook and you're not going to be quizzed on this, but let's do a quick timeline of the history of sleep study and discoveries in the last century:

1903—Dr. Emil Fischer and physician Josef von Mering created the sleeping pill barbital, the precursor to barbiturates.

1911—Dr. Henri Piéron found that sleep-deprived animals had "some sort of a" chemical in their cerebrospinal fluid that when injected into alert dogs made them fall asleep, which is most likely a very early (and unbeknownst) trial on melatonin.

1916—Physician Constantin von Economo credited the hypothalamus as being responsible for wakefulness and sleep.

1925—Nathaniel Kleitman began studying REM sleep, cognition, and sleep deprivation.

1956—Professor Charles Sidney Burwell identified the condition now known as obstructive sleep apnea.

1958—Dr. Aaron Lerner discovered melatonin, the hormone responsible for regulating sleep-wake cycles.

1968—Professor Allan Rechtschaffen and Dr. Anthony Kales published the first guideline for determining sleep stages. This guide is still used today to define the four non-REM stages of sleep according to brain wave patterns.

1970—Dr. William Dement founded the first sleep lab, at Stanford University, specifically focused on studying sleep disorders.

1973—Professor Thomas Borkovec conducted cognitive behavioral therapy studies for insomnia.

1975—The Association of Sleep Disorders Centers, which later became the American Academy of Sleep Medicine (AASM), was founded.

1975—Dr. William Dement and Dr. Mary Carskadon created the multiple sleep latency test, which helps diagnose a variety of sleep disorders.

1977—Dr. Peter Hauri published a guideline for sleep hygiene.

1980—Dr. Colin Sullivan developed the continuous positive airway pressure (CPAP) system for treating sleep apnea.

1982—Dr. Carlyle Smith researched rats and found that REM sleep is imperative to learning and recollection.

Alright, so now you're caught up. But there's a huge disconnect between almost all sleep research conducted up until recently, and human optimization, especially when it comes to sports. Most sleep research has been conducted on psychological factors and how they relate to the human condition or even some cognitive functions—learning, mood, dreams, etc. What sleep researchers haven't focused on is the link between sleep and physiological human functions—that's really all I care about, and if you're reading this book, it should be of interest to you too!

HUSH LITTLE BABY

For any of you parents out there, you already know most of this next part, even if you don't know you do, or what it actually means.

Babies sleep a lot. They need their sleep . . . a lot. And old people wake up, drink their coffee, go fishing—twice—and make breakfast for the family, all before the moody teenager comes out to wage war on everyone within a two-mile vicinity. That's not an individual discrepancy. It's not random. It's pretty darn universal. And there's a biological reason for that. What do you notice from the chart below from the Sleep Study Foundation?

BLOOM'S TAXONOMY		
Infant	4–12 months	12–16 hours (including naps)
Toddler	1–2 years	11–14 hours (including naps)
Preschool	3–5 years	10–13 hours (including naps)
School-age	6–12 years	9–12 hours
Teen	13–18 years	8–10 hours
Adult	18 years and older	7 hours or more

Infants and newborns get more than twice the amount of sleep as adults. It's not a coincidence that the amount of development during each phase corresponds with the amount of sleep needed during that time period. Sleep is essential for growth. When we are infants, the body physically has to grow. When we are toddlers, the brain is developing so much with language; toddlers see abstract thought for the first time and really begin to learn in social settings. During puberty, the reproductive organs become pronounced and functional, and there is also more complex brain development.

But as we get into adulthood, we forget about this process because we don't see the changes. And sleep for development really becomes sleep for recovery. Just because we don't need more sleep for development, that doesn't mean we can operate on less and less sleep.

If we just think about it for a quick moment—if all of that development throughout our life occurs when we sleep, why do we think it's any different as adults when we work out hard? When we study hard? When we're exposed to bacteria and viruses? Just like in bodybuilding and powerlifting, there's a saying, "the gains are made in the recovery." Well, SLEEP IS THE RECOVERY! It doesn't matter if it's mental recovery or physical recovery, sleep is where the body repairs itself—in a million different ways!

As adults, we no longer need sleep for development. We need it to maintain. We need it to perform!

DIGGING DEEPER

So what happens during sleep? We know we dream, but other than that, it just seems like nothingness. I'd always thought when I slept without remembering dreams, it was the closest state imaginable to death. The absence of consciousness. The absence of thought.

For as long as I can remember, I've hated sleep. The lack of something to me is reprehensible. I would go to sleep in a hurry to wake up, so I could do . . . anything. So I could produce. The same way I can't sit down and relax because there are things to be done is the same way I go to sleep wanting to wake up. I love the day. I love being able to work. And I love coffee. I've always been the guy burning the candle at both ends. Go on as little sleep as possible. Look what I can do. Look how much stuff I can get done in a day while you sleep. But now, as I look further and further into sleep, as I look further and further into the ailments I've gone through over the years—especially as the magic of my youth dissipated—I realize sleep is actually the closest thing to immortality we have. It's more similar to our days in the womb than our days in the grave.

WHY, THOUGH?

As I said earlier, all the real building occurs during sleep. If the body is a house, and we don't want our house to become unlivable and dilapidated, there must be constant upkeep. If the roof needs to be replaced, well, first the old roof needs to be removed. If the tile is out of style, it must be removed before new flooring can be installed. Think of daytime as the breakdown process—we lift weights, which breaks down our muscles. We use our brain, which drains our mental battery. During sleep is when the new roof and flooring are installed. During sleep is when our muscles are rebuilt and our brains are cleansed of toxins and by-products. Sleep is when the body does all its best repair work. But just like different phases during building a house—foundation, framing, finish—there are phases of sleep, and they each have a very specific purpose and role.

BREAKING IT DOWN

You might think we'd categorize the phases of sleep based on what occurs within the body during each phase, but we don't. We label each based on the type of brain waves elicited during each phase. Sleep isn't induced by the body. The body doesn't call for sleep. The brain does. And that's why we categorize the phases of sleep based on the brain activity and brain waves that occur during each phase. The brain induces sleep by secreting GABA (gamma-aminobutyric acid) and melatonin based on the body's circadian rhythm. Then, the brain sends out signals for each phase of sleep that directs the body to react and perform in a very specific manner during each phase.

There are four phases of sleep broken down into two major categories: rapid eye movement sleep and non-rapid eye movement sleep. The four phases are non-REM sleep 1 (NREM 1), non-REM sleep 2 (NREM 2), non-REM sleep 3 (NREM 3), and REM sleep. Although not very different in name, they are, indeed, very different in bodily function.

Overall, people spend about 75–90% in non-REM sleep, and 10–25% in REM sleep. Furthermore, we spend approximately 5% of our sleep in NREM 1; approximately 50% in NREM 2; 20% in NREM 3 (deep sleep); and 25% in REM sleep. As we age, we spend less and less time in NREM 3, which may very well be cause for significant physical decline as we grow older.

NREM 1

NREM 1 is the first stage of sleep, but it's more of the pathway to sleep than an actual sleep stage. It's the wormhole between two dimensions: awake and sleeping. When normal to optimal sleeping conditions are met, this is generally when the heart rate and breathing slow down. Muscles begin to relax, and brain waves slow. Lower frequency waves are being produced by the brain, but they're higher theta waves—something you'd experience during drowsiness or daydreaming. They're not the low frequency waves seen in deep sleep—still high enough to cause a muscle spasm as your body is figuring out just what parts to close up shop for the night, but not high enough for conscious thought or conscious muscle action.

When normal to optimal measures are not met for NREM 1 stage of sleep, traveling through the consciousness wormhole from awake to sleep will be difficult. These un-ideal conditions could be caused by a plethora of reasons. Being on your phone (certain lights) is going to change the body's circadian rhythm and slow the release of melatonin, keeping the brain more active, for one common example. But there are a hundred examples of poor sleep habits that will disrupt this stage. Working out too close to bedtime. Drinking caffeine too late in the day. Eating certain foods or eating too close (or early) to bedtime. Alcohol consumption. Drug use—even marijuana, or over-the-counter medications (different people are sensitive to different compounds and this is all subjective). And maybe the worst culprit of them all, stress! Stress can keep your brain active. It can increase your heart rate. Cause pain and discomfort. Stress can kill your sleep quality fast, and miserably.

But all these habits can lead to a change in brain activity, heart rate, breathing, and countless other physiological changes that can affect sleep in a negative or positive way.

Sleep is a state set off by the brain. The brain needs to slow down to create the optimal sleep environment, and when the brain is active due to outside stressors (thinking of work, relationships, etc.) it has a much more difficult time inducing the proper environment to go through the sleep portal.

NREM 2

When you come out the other side of the consciousness wormhole, you find yourself in NREM 2—actual sleep. During NREM 2 the body temperature continues to cool, blood pressure decreases, the heart rate slows, and muscles begin to relax more. Although NREM 2 is not the deepest phase of the sleep cycle, it is still very restful and restorative. But the real defining characteristic of NREM 2 is the presence of sleep spindles, a type of brain wave that is important in memory and motor function learning. As the sleep cycle progresses throughout the night, more time is spent in this phase than any other.

There's a new trend in learning that involves naps. As a napper myself, I don't need an extra reason, but I'll take it. Go listen to Dr. Andrew Huberman, and he'll mention naps after learning a thousand times. So, how does this occur? I'm no neuroscientist and you're not in need of a neuroscience book, but the very short version is that sleep spindles and NREM 2 sleep help not only process memories from the short term to the long term (intellect), but they also help implant motor skills from the short term (practiced) to the long term (physical skills and muscle memory).

The famed neuroscientist Dr. Matthew Walker, years before he wrote his bestselling book *Why We Sleep,* wrote an article titled "Practice with Sleep Makes Perfect: Sleep-Dependent Motor Skill Learning." In a meta-analysis of sleep articles, Walker came across a study where sixty-two participants were tested on "finger tapping tasks," a motor skill—think of playing the guitar or piano—that's a mix of cognitive function and motor-function (very similar to athletic skills vs just learning information such as math or language). The participants were tested at either 10 AM or 10 PM. Those tested at 10 AM were retested again in four-hour increments (2 PM, 6 PM, 10 PM). There was no significant difference between the test results at the 10 AM practice/test session and the test 12 hours later. However, those tested at 10 PM were subsequently tested again 12 hours later, after a night of sleep, and the average increase in test score was 18.9%. For doing nothing. Just sleeping in between sessions, and an 18.9% increase occurred.

The NREM 2 sleep is paramount for learning and processing both motor and intellectual information, and I'd suggest any time you want to learn a new language or study for that test, or work a new crossover in basketball, you go home and take a nap. The great thing about NREM 2 is you can reach that phase with a "power nap," as it's a lighter phase of sleep, whereas trying to get into NREM 3 will take a much longer time to access. Sleep isn't just recharging your batteries, it's transferring the data from the SD card onto the computer hard drive for you to access at a later date.

If sleep is a "super drug," think of this phase as the "limitless" pill from the 2011 Bradley Cooper movie. This is the pill giving him the super brainpower to achieve the great heights of his personal computing power.

NREM 3

If NREM 2 is the "brain" sleep, NREM 3 is the "body" sleep.

This phase is considered "deep sleep" and accounts for approximately 20–25% of the sleep cycle. More time is spent here earlier in the night/sleep cycle, and the time spent here decreases throughout the night and may disappear altogether toward the last sleep cycle. Most of the physical rebuilding process occurs during this sleep stage. That makes sense if you think about it. During NREM 3, the body is at its lowest resting metabolic rate (calories burned while resting) during the 24(ish) hours of the body's circadian rhythm. The brain is transmitting slow wave synchronization (SWS) brain waves and is using less energy. The heart rate slows further. Blood pressure drops to a 24-hour low. Muscles are relaxed. During this time when the body expends so little energy, it is able to use that energy to release the body's inflammatory response to fight off bacteria and viruses and repair muscles and tissues. During NREM 3 testosterone and human growth hormone are secreted, aiding in muscle and tissue repair.

In terms of pure physicality, this is the sleep stage you want to be in. When adequate amounts of sleep in this stage occur, there are different hormones secreted that affect physical appearance (belly fat) and musculature.

Leptin and ghrelin help regulate hunger and calorie burn. Leptin is a hormone that tells your body whether you are hungry or not and when to burn calories. Ghrelin gives the body the "full" feeling after eating. If your sleep habits are flipped upside down, the hormone telling you you're not hungry and the hormone telling you you're full aren't produced. And you wonder why the medical community says chronic sleep deprivation can lead to weight gain and has links to diabetes? If you're an athlete who needs to stay within the confines of a certain body fat percentage or a weight class, good luck keeping the weight off when you're not sleeping well.

Cortisol is also heavily secreted during this phase, which is the stress hormone, or the body's inflammatory response to stress. Cortisol increases during this phase so cytokines and other anti-viral/anti-bacterial immune responses can keep the body free of attackers. Cortisol levels rise during the night and lower during waking hours. And although short-term sleep disturbances won't necessarily affect cortisol levels, chronic sleep disturbances may lead to increased cortisol during the daytime—which can cause chronic high blood pressure, increased blood glucose levels, an increase in weight, and possibly diabetes.

And, of course, the good stuff: HGH and testosterone. Both of these hormones are highest during NREM 3 phases of sleep, and if that sleep period is disrupted, both decline. In fact, 70% of the body's HGH is created during NREM 3 sleep!

It's no wonder, as we get older, we spend less and less time in NREM 3 sleep and more and more time in REM and NREM 2 sleep, which perfectly correlates with our reduction in HGH and testosterone production—which greatly correlates with our ability (or inability) to produce/grow lean muscle mass and burn fat.

REM

REM sleep, or Rapid Eye Movement sleep, has traditionally been the focus of sleep for millennia. Sigmund Freud wrote *The Interpretation of Dreams* in 1900 and founded an entire psychological practice on the subject. But the analysis and interpretation of dreams has been going on since the beginning of time. In the book of Genesis alone, there are countless references to dreams and their interpretations and meanings. And yet, we know so little about them. What they mean. Why we have them. How they occur.

What we do know about REM sleep is that each cycle can last between 10 minutes and 1 hour, and typically increases in length later in the sleep cycle. The time we spend in REM tends to decline with age. The brain waves emitted during REM are more closely related to those seen when we are awake, and our blood pressure, body temperature, and heart rate rise to near-awake levels. Our bodies go into a physical paralysis during this sleep phase, which is most likely a defense mechanism so you don't act out the dreams in real life.

Some medical practitioners believe REM is used as an "unlearning" process for the brain—similar to clearing a computer's hard drive so new information can be introduced and stored. Others believe this is the phase of sleep that is responsible for cleaning out the waste buildup of the brain's processing power throughout the day.

Oddly enough, as fascinating as this stage is, we don't seem to need it much at all. Many people who are on SSRIs for depression have significantly reduced time in REM sleep, or even zero time spent in the phase, and there don't seem to be any detrimental responses to the lack of the phase.

Lastly, animals dream too. That is something we do know, and there are even reports that dogs dream of their owners. So, whatever is going on seems to be a mammalian biological process that goes beyond just human cognition.

Famed sleep expert Dr. Matthew Walker writes in his bestseller *Why We Sleep* about how the advent of dreaming may be what pushed us on the evolutionary ladder higher than other living creatures.

WHEN WE DON'T SLEEP

You're not here for a sleep education, though, and you want to know "why should I care?" And let me tell you, there're a lot of reasons to care. On just a normal, human function level of operating, well, sleep deprivation has been linked to numerous chronic health conditions like heart disease, kidney disease, high blood pressure, diabetes, stroke, depression, and obesity.

Now that we got that out of the way, why you're here: you want to perform better. Whether it's for sport, physical looks, or optimizing performance in some way. And let me tell you, I've seen sleep deprivation ruin more dreams than virtually every other roadblock combined.

One of the worst feelings as an athlete is when you're mid–training camp, and things seem to be clicking. You're feeling stronger. You're feeling faster. Winning more practice races and sparring rounds. Hitting PRs (personal records). You're beginning to think you're unstoppable. And then you hit a wall of sickness, or worse, injury.

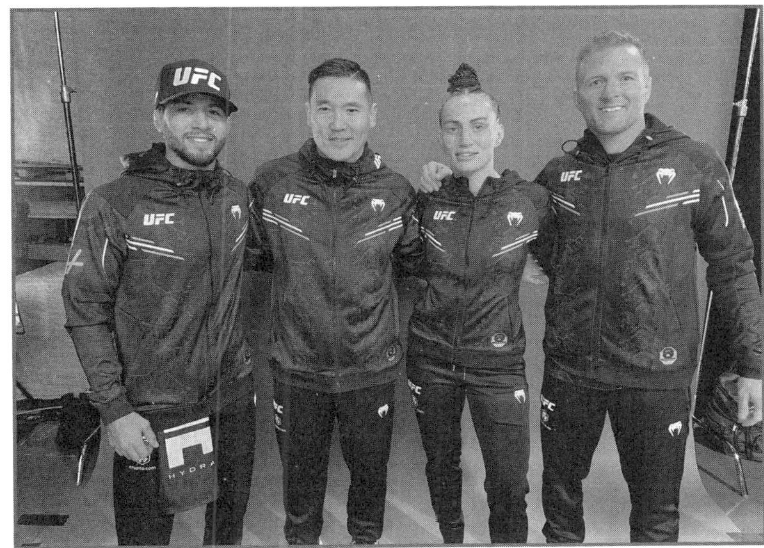

Casey O'Neill is one of the hardest workers I've ever met, but too much work and not enough rest have led to injuries for her. *Seigher Brown*

SLEEP AND THE IMMUNE SYSTEM

It happened to me. It could happen to you.

I am naturally a stressed-out human. I'm type A. I wake up and drink three to four cups of coffee before I leave my house. I'm always operating at a high level, and the thought of underperforming for even a few hours is a nightmare. I don't relax. I don't have hobbies. When I have free time, I work—writing, editing videos, watching film on my fighter's MMA opponents. That's what I consider fun. The closest thing I do that others would consider relaxing is reading. My time on this earth is limited. Can't waste any. I'd probably be considered ADHD if I were to see a psychologist/medical professional, but I don't feel like it's affecting my life negatively, so I don't see the need. Years ago, though, it may have very well been the underlying cause of major recurring staph infections.

If you've spent much time around sports—which I'm assuming you have, since you're reading this book—you've seen, or at least heard of, a multitude of skin infections. There's ringworm. A fungal infection that takes the shape of a round, raised formation on the skin. It may be as small as a bug bite, or may cover an entire back, face, or arm. I've even seen ringworm on the scalp, and as disgusting as it is, on the tongue. Then, there's herpes—not the mouth or sexually transmitted version, but skin (or "mat") herpes, which can be either herpes simplex 1 or simplex 2 (which are actually the same as mouth/genital herpes, but transmitted through skin-to-skin contact, not sexually). It may be hard to discern from staph or impetigo or even fungal infections. Sometimes herpes gets misdiagnosed as a bacterial infection that won't go away for weeks. Those affected by herpes will usually feel a tingling sensation in the area a day or so prior to an outbreak. Outbreaks are usually painful but may also itch/burn as well. If left untreated, outbreaks will generally clear up in approximately two weeks, though with medication, may go away in a day or so. One huge cause of herpes outbreaks is stress—athletic training camps are generally very full of stress: emotional stress, training load stress, financial stress; add lack of sleep to the mix, and . . . well we'll get more into herpes later. But herpes isn't the last of the skin infections, and certainly not the worst. There's staph infections.

Staph has countless different strains and manifests in a myriad of different ways. Some have rash-looking infections. Others have boils and abscesses. While others manifest as blisters on the head and neck with yellow/orange ooze dripping out in the form of impetigo. Staph is gross. It may hurt. It may itch. It may burn. But worst of all, it may mutate. Don't take my word for it. A quick Google search will show you everything you never wanted to see.

Traditionally, most staph infections were treated with methicillin antibiotics. You've probably had amoxicillin in your lifetime for a toothache or strep throat. However, through the overprescribing and overuse of methicillin drugs, staph has become resistant to those antibiotics, which has brought about the "super bacteria" MRSA (methicillin-resistant Staphylococcus aureus). Staph infections have sent many, many people to the hospital, and MRSA has said, "Hold my beer" and wreaked havoc on countless individuals, often leading to hospitalizations, amputations, sepsis, and even death. But I digress.

In my early thirties, I was getting staph infections too often. Most people go their entire life avoiding a staph infection. I was getting them three, four, five times a year. When I was on the UFC show *The Ultimate Fighter*, I spent almost the entire six and a half weeks of filming on antibiotics for a staph infection. I was given methicillin antibiotics and the infection got worse and worse for days on end. I told producers, but they told me the antibiotics take time to work. Eventually, I threw a fit and screamed and threatened every human I could, and they took me back to the doctor, where I received IV antibiotics twice a week, in addition to the two oral antibiotics I was prescribed for the remainder of the show. Years later, and I was getting the infections again. At one point, I was prescribed doxycycline for sixty days straight, as my dermatologist thought MRSA bacteria was living in my sinuses, and they had to nuke my entire body to get rid of it all.

It always happened the same way: I'd train hard for a few days in a row. Then I wouldn't sleep well for a day or so. Keep training hard. Staph. Rinse repeat. Sometimes it would start with me not sleeping well for a few days. Then I'd train. Staph. Other times I would feel a scratch in my throat. "Am I getting sick?" I'd ask. Train. Not sleep well for a day or so. Staph.

This occurred on and off for years. My wife was getting nervous. I was getting nervous. "If you get staph one more time, you're going to have to quit training fighters. This is bad," she said. I knew she was right. How many doses of Bactrim could I take before it just didn't work on me anymore? Then what, I get a simple infection and have no way to eradicate it? What's the end game?

Then, fortuitously, I found myself in the office of Dr. Roman Fomin, the chief science director of the UFC Performance Institute—a facility owned and operated by the UFC to give UFC fighters the greatest care in sports performance.

We were there to discuss one of my fighters at the time, Frankie Saenz, a bantamweight in the UFC. We'd just finished a workout, and Roman began hooking Frankie up to electrodes similar to an EKG machine. There were a few on his chest. One on his hand and two on his head.

"Now I want you to lie down there on the floor and relax, Frankie. Just focus on your breathing, and tune me and Santino out. Try not to focus on home or your fight or anything stressful. Just let your mind drift," he said in a thick Russian accent.

As Roman and I spoke, we monitored Frankie's heart rate and brain waves. His heart rate was in the eighties, as he'd just finished a workout. More interestingly, his brain waves were shooting up and down. Large, long strokes of an active mind. Roman and I continued talking and eventually, around five minutes after Frankie lay down, his brain waves crashed and began to go up and down very slowly. He'd found a way to turn off his brain. Within a few seconds of his brain calming down, his heart rate dropped. Seventy-five beats. Then seventy. Sixty. And so on.

"You see, the brain can't focus on the body when it's focused on the brain," Roman said. "The brain takes a lot of energy to stay active. But when the brain calms down, the body calms down. Because the brain can send all that brain energy to recovery for the body."

And that was the start of me tracking my vitals and recovery. I bought a Polar watch that tracked my sleep, HRV (heart rate variability—we'll get more into this later), heart rate, and overall recovery. I became obsessed with my recovery score. But I noticed the largest indicator of my recovery and whether I was ready to push the next day had to do with two things. The first was how hard I trained the day before, and the second, my sleep score. Almost overnight, I focused on optimizing my sleep. If I ate too close to bedtime, my sleep would suffer. Drink alcohol? My score tanked. Even a single drink would drop my sleep score significantly, but I noticed whiskey or hard liquor hurt it more than a beer. Stressed out? Forget about it. Tanked.

Eventually, I figured it out, though. I learned what would allow me to sleep well and what would create a poor sleep score. And as my sleep quality continued to go up and up, the time I spent sick or with staph infections dropped and dropped. I now consider myself superior to most humans in regard to my immune system. I rarely get sick. I haven't gotten staph in nearly a decade. Even during the height of the Covid-19 pandemic, I avoided the virus for over a year. I'd be training alongside fighters who were dropping left and right from Covid, and I stood on my island of immunity alone. I'd train with them one day; the next, they'd be sick. Yet I avoided the sickness. I now find myself sick once every two to three years, and rarely worry about becoming ill or contracting skin infections.

In the third phase of NREM sleep, the body's inflammatory response rises, allowing for cytokines and T cells to get to work fighting viruses and bacterial infiltrators. This stage alone may be the very most important time of the day for the immune system's ability to stave off attackers and maintain its health.

WANT TO SEE AN INJURED ATHLETE?

Sleep-deprived athletes face a 1.7 times greater risk of being injured than those who receive adequate sleep

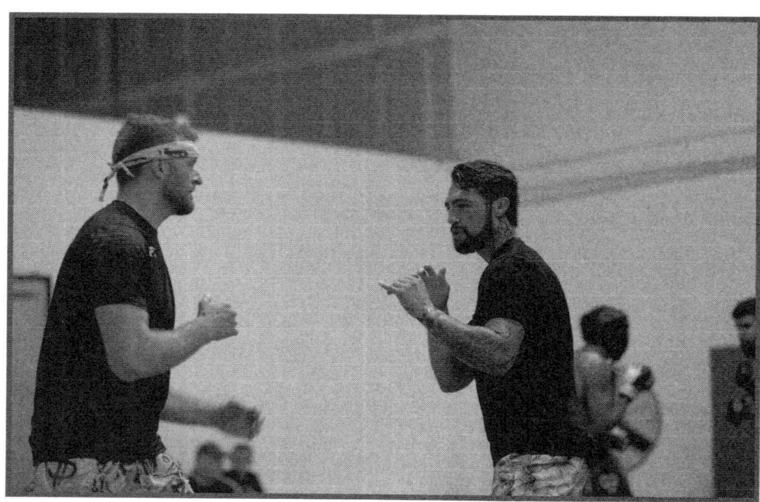

Before his 30th birthday, Kameula Kirk had over 10 surgeries. He is the most injury-plagued fighter I know, and also has the worst sleep schedule. *Seigher Brown*

One of the most common things I hear with my fighters is, "I didn't sleep well last night" (or for the last few nights). It doesn't even shock me anymore. I don't ask questions like I used to. "Do you feel sick?" "Are you stressed?" "Have you been on your phone late?" Those used to be the questions I'd ask. Now, almost always, it's not a question I'm asking, but a statement I'm making. "You're overtraining." Nobody wants to hear it. Nobody wants to take time off as a competition nears. But poor sleep or insomnia are telltale signs of overtraining. However, there's a bit of a chicken and the egg situation to deal with between sleep and overtraining and poor recovery. Poor sleep leads to overtraining, as the muscles can't be repaired due to the lack of sleep, but overtraining also leads to sleep disruption, which, in turn, leads to poor recovery and the body going down a slippery slope of a cycle spiraling out of control. As the days of pushing the physical limits mount, while sleep decreases, the overtraining pressure builds and builds until something ruptures—generally an ACL in the knee is what that rupture is, but either way, an injury forces the brakes to be pumped.

HOW DOES SLEEP DEPRIVATION LEAD TO INJURIES?

It would be nice if I told you sleep deprivation did one specific thing that causes injuries, and then you could say, "Well, I'll combat that with X." But I can't do that because, just like everything in the body, it doesn't work that way. There's a myriad of organs and processes swirling around at all times in the body that create homeostasis, just as there's not one gene expression in our DNA that makes us tall or fast or susceptible to asthma. And, like so many other areas with our body, with athletic performance, and with human existence (what's the meaning of life?), we just don't have all the answers. But I, for one, am somewhat okay with not having the answers, and I certainly am not going to make stuff up or create connections between anything just to make you feel better. The good news, though, is we know enough about sleep and how it affects our bodies to list various effects of poor sleep—now, how much weight do we place on each of them for injuries? Well, I'd probably have an easier time explaining the purpose of human life than that.

Cognitive function: Sleep deprivation leads to reduced cognition. You know that. I know that. We've heard it from the beginning of grade school. "Get a good night's rest before the test." It's not new. It's hard to learn when we haven't slept, and it's hard to recall learned information when we're tired too.

We sometimes forget, though, that athletics use our brains just as much (if not more) than academics. Reaction time, decision-making, cognition are all used in athletics—especially in tennis, golf, and combat sports. Accuracy declines when we're tired, which is needed for golf, tennis, basketball, combat sports. We need our brains to be as sharp as we would want them for a test while we're on the free throw line or the balance beam. Could you imagine being a wide receiver in the NFL and your quarterback calls for a play with an out-route in the end zone, but you get the plays mixed up and run a go route? Brains matter in sports. Well-functioning brains win. Our brains have to be firing on all cylinders to excel, but they also need to be running well in the background so as to not fail at a basic level. Slipping a punch to the left or the right may be the difference in winning a boxing fight or waking up looking up at the lights asking, "What happened?"

When the fog of sleep deprivation clouds our reflexes, it may cause overcompensation of movements, which we all know can lead to injuries. If we're on the tennis court, we expect the ball to be hit near the service line, but if it goes farther toward the baseline than we expected, we have to change our reaction times and our exertion level, and our body may pull a muscle or tear a ligament because of the change in speed or effort. If you're an athlete, you know about thinking you were "good" in a situation (thought you were wide open, thought you were safe from a punch or kick), but then there was a change in what you perceived to be the case, causing you to fail in that moment (being taken down in wrestling, missing the ball in the end zone). And we all know the same scenario that, instead of causing a failure in those moments, caused an injury—we were going light, but then he picked up the pace or I slipped up, and I got hurt. Sleep deprivation and cognition play a role in that reaction time, but aren't the sole culprit!

Glycogen: In simple terms, we use glycogen for energy expenditure during most anaerobic AND aerobic activity. When we don't sleep well, we don't break down and store as much glycogen as we do on a full night's rest. During aerobic work, the cardiovascular system is also used to transport glycogen and oxygen to muscles during workouts, which may also be inhibited due to the lack of sleep—further inhibiting the body's full use of glycogen for athletic workloads. And, again, there's not a clear path as to "why does limiting muscle glycogen play a role in sleep deprivation and athletic injuries," but if we look at everything holistically, we can see that having less energy in one system could lead to the overreaching of another system while trying to compensate. Tired, fatigued quads and hamstrings due to the lack of energy stores while trying to cut during a football route could place too much stress on the ACL. Not having the energy to jump as high on a pole vault might lead to overarching the back. There are direct and indirect ways injuries may occur.

Inflammation (the bad kind): We talked about inflammation's role in the immune system as cytokines are released that help fight off bacteria and viruses, but inflammation in the body should rise during sleep and subside as you wake. That's the normal, healthy cycle. There's also a natural occurrence of acute inflammation when you injure yourself. Roll an ankle or bump your knee, and you'll see it balloon up almost immediately. That's also a natural, good type of inflammation. It starts the body's healing process, and the inflammation (fluid) also serves as a buffer to shield the bone or injured area from other harmful bumps and abrasions. It's like football pads for your hurt body part.

Now, I said I wasn't going to draw too many conclusions to answers that we don't have a full, clear picture of. We don't exactly know if chronic inflammation causes or correlates with injuries perfectly. What we do know is that chronic inflammation wreaks havoc on the body, and its levels rise significantly with sleep deprivation and, as mentioned before, chronic inflammation can lead to high blood pressure, diabetes, heart disease, depression, anxiety, and scores of other ailments—disassociating the body from homeostasis. And for the body to perform optimally, we'd expect the need for a homeostatic baseline to handle the stresses and needs of high-level athletics.

But going back to the acute inflammation of the injured area. We want that inflammation to be present for a short period of time—long enough to repair the injured area of our body, and then that needs to go. If we have too much chronic inflammation, that may change the acute inflammation and cause it to go away too soon or stay for too long, which in itself can change the body's way of handling running and turns and physical movements. If a swollen knee is bothering a runner, the body will compensate by putting more weight on the opposite knee or ankle or lower back. The body wants to be efficient and pain free, and it will always compensate as it sees fit—but not always generating long-term positive results.

Testosterone: We can all do steroids if we sleep better. Testosterone is the male sex hormone, and one of the major hormones our body produces while we sleep. During in-utero development, and in the presence of the Y chromosome, it signals the male genitalia to form. During puberty, it's responsible for further sex organ development, bone density, lean muscle mass growth, facial hair growth. In short, it's what makes men . . . men. As a performance enhancer, athletes have injected testosterone (usually synthetic) to aid in the repair of muscle tissues postworkout and to aid in overall recovery. But, just as with human growth hormone, testosterone is predominantly synthesized in the body during sleep—and is highest in the bloodstream during the early morning hours, after a good night's sleep. And if you're not sleeping, you're not producing testosterone at the same level as your dreaming peers. Not only are you missing out on the gains attributed to testosterone, but you may even be running at a deficit if your body isn't able to repair torn muscle fibers caused by the rigorous workload of athletics.

Growth hormone: Just as it sounds, human growth hormone initiates growth and repair in virtually every cell in the body. Produced by the pituitary gland in the brain and regulated by hormones produced in the brain, stomach, and pancreas, HGH is almost exclusively produced during the NREM 3 phase of sleep. HGH is thought to contribute to the reduction of fat in adults and denser bones. Repairing and maintaining cartilage are among its other benefits. Many athletes and bodybuilders credit testosterone with helping build muscle, and HGH to helping keep joints, ligaments, and cartilage healthy. But one of the circular benefits attributed to HGH treatment in adults is better sleep. When HGH is higher, sleep tends to be better. When sleep is better, the body tends to produce more HGH. Now, I'm not suggesting any form of supplementation (that's for you to discuss with a medical professional), but it seems logical that the sleep-to-HGH production cycle would be best maintained through regular good sleeping habits.

We don't know all of the nuanced positive effects of HGH on the body, but we know levels are much higher during youth and peak during puberty. Children tend to bounce back from injury so much faster than adults without the need for surgery. Joints expand. Bones grow. Cells repair quickly. If HGH is the fountain of youth Dorian Gray sought, sleep deprivation and the lack of HGH production is the painting growing old on the mantel.

TIME TO DO SOMETHING ABOUT IT: HOW TO OPTIMIZE YOUR SLEEP

Identifying a problem is the first step in solving a problem, but with your poor sleep habits, you may have to dig deeper and identify numerous side-quest problems as well. You know you're not getting the sleep you need, but what's the cause? I doubt it's just one. Is it the blue light emitting from your phone? The alcohol? Stress? It's all of the above, but good sleep starts long before you climb into bed and close your eyes. It starts before the day even begins. It starts with good habits.

Let's go through the usual suspects of poor sleep.

1. Build good habits. The three good habits that I recommend to everyone are to go to sleep at the same (relative) time every night, only use your bed for sleep (and sex), and don't bring your phone into the bedroom. I don't even charge my phone at night in my room. It stays in the office and charges away from me.

    A. Going to sleep every night at the same time helps your body's circadian rhythm set a fixed schedule, which is going to aid in the production of GABA and melatonin at the right time to send you off to your zzz's. It also has numerous health benefits, such as decreased risk of cardiovascular disease, increased learning among children compared to those who went to bed at any time (even when they got enough sleep), and decreased behavioral and mood issues amongst children and teens.

    B. If you only use your bed for sleep and sex, you train your body to sleep. It's like Pavlov's dog experiment with a bed. However, if you're used to watching TV, playing video games, or working on your laptop, your brain won't be trained to slow down when it's bedtime. Offices are for work. Living rooms are for TV and games. Bedrooms are for sleep.

C. And phones . . . oh boy, phones! Not only should phones not be in the bedroom, as they keep your brain stimulated, they should be avoided for a few hours leading up to bedtime to limit the blue light, which the body reads as sunlight and which inhibits the production of melatonin and GABA.

2. If habits is step one, done long before you sleep, two through twenty-seven are all PUT YOUR DAMN PHONE DOWN, but for brevity, we'll keep it at just two. Your phone is killing your sleep.

3. Wind down. You need to take some time before you go to bed—approximately thirty minutes or so—to begin the sleep process. Don't rush around. Get the house in order. Ready the next day's work or school—get clothes out, pack your lunch, ready any materials you know you need. And then put on comfy clothes, put the snacks down, and brush your teeth. Get a little bored. And, again, get rid of that phone.

4. Slow your brain down and de-stress and de-digitize. One of the biggest issues people have with getting to sleep is the racing thoughts of the mind. You have that big sales meeting tomorrow. You have a test. You've been fighting with your girlfriend. Try to organize all of the worries that are going through your head. Anxiety is created by worrying about things we can't control, so worry about the things you CAN control—and handle them! Make a checklist of what you need done—in your personal life (do you go to bed late and drink too much?), in your financial life (do you have bills that need to be paid?), and of course in your training life (were you

supposed to run earlier for your cardio? Did you skip a meal or eat too much?) Handle your life, and check things off your to-do list. Procrastination leads to anxiety, and anxiety leads to restless nights and a racing mind. If your life isn't in order outside of the sport, it's not going to magically fix itself during training or while competing.

Another way I like to slow my brain is through reading books. I've noticed that when I'm reading before bed (or regularly for that matter), I am waaay less "ADHD." My brain slows down. I don't crave social media as much. I'm less agitated. Books are soothing to my brain, and I bet they'd do yours a world of good too—you're reading this, so you're good!

5. Track what you put in your body. I know when I eat too close to bedtime, I don't sleep well. But if I'm hungry, I won't sleep well either! There's a balance. Even a glass of alcohol near bedtime, and my sleep is trash, but if I have a drink around 5 PM or earlier, it doesn't affect me as much. White wine and sparkling wine affect me the least. Red wine or any sort of hard alcohol affects me the most. Everyone is different, so you need to keep a log of these things, which brings me to my next point.

6. Keep a sleep log. Write down what you ate and the time. What you drank. Did you have alcohol? Marijuana or other drugs? Did you eat, and at what time? Does a bowl of cereal affect you differently than popcorn or ice cream or chicken?

7. Manage the temperature. It's not always feasible to regulate the room temperature, as some people don't have central AC, while

others don't have heat—or worse, your partner likes the bedroom hot or hates the cost of an overused air conditioning bill. But find the temperature that works best for you and track that in your log. Generally speaking, cooler temperatures produce better sleep. These temps vary, but anywhere between 68- and 74-degrees Fahrenheit tends to be better than warm temperatures. It makes sense, as our natural body temperature drops while we sleep. We want to be cold.

8. Another overlooked sleep aid is the materials you're actually sleeping on. Invest in the absolute best bed you can afford. You'll pay that extra money for the nicer car, but you won't pay an extra two hundred dollars on a bed? You spend a third of your life in that thing, buy a good one. And while you're at it, get some thousand-thread-count Egyptian cotton sheets and a nice pillow too. It will change your life.

9. Eyeshades and earplugs aren't just for the airplane. If you have light seeping into your room, or maybe a partner who wakes up early or turns the light on when going to the bathroom during the night, you may want to try an eye shade—yup, those silly eye covers you see people in the movies put on. Keeping your eyes hidden from unwanted light will definitely help you maintain a better sleep pattern. So will earplugs. My life CHANGED when I started wearing earplugs to sleep. I never realized how much ambient noise kept my brain on alert and running in the background. When I plug my ears before bed, I sleep infinitely better.

10. Wearables—usually watches or some sort of strap or ring that tracks your sleep and recovery. I'll talk about wearables more later. There are so many on the market these days (Apple watch, Polar, Fitbit, Garmin, Whoop, Oura Ring, and more), and each has its own niche for consumers, but they can also be a crutch and lead to diminishing returns.

3

TECHNIQUE IS CRITICAL

There are no shortcuts when it comes to perfecting the intricacies of fight craft. And even the best, most naturally gifted fighters sometimes need to return to the basics. Not all fighters have the same strengths, of course, but in a sport where one wrong move can get you knocked out (or worse), fighters who are technically precise and consistent in that precision will make fewer mistakes and, in turn, give themselves the best chance to win. In this chapter I will run through technical workouts with a number of elite fighters to demonstrate how being fundamentally sound and in control, physically and mentally, provides fighters with the ability to execute their fight plan confidently and without hesitation.

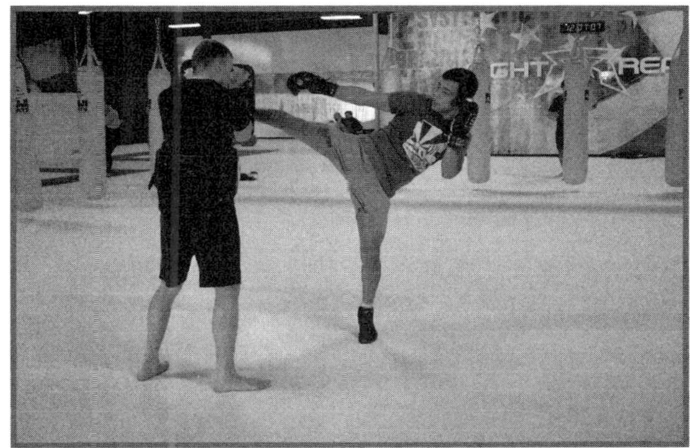

Here I work with Christian Rodriguez as we try to touch on details with his kicks.

Seigher Brown

I tell my fighters all the time that winning and losing in the cage isn't about who's better. It's about who messes up first. And generally speaking, the fighter who is going to mess up first is the one who either has faulty fundamentals or worse cardio (which we'll discuss later). Everybody is really fast and athletic in round one. So if you throw a jab at me and I'm athletic, I can just get out of the way of it. That jab isn't going to land. But as the fight wears on and I start to slow down, my athleticism won't be enough to keep me upright if my opponent is more technically sound than I am, especially if I've got to make big dynamic movements to avoid getting hit or getting taken down. If, however, I am more economical in my movements—i.e., more technical—it won't be nearly as exhausting. And when a fighter's athleticism starts to slip a little bit, their speed and ability to move slip as well.

At that point, it's all fundamentals. All technique.

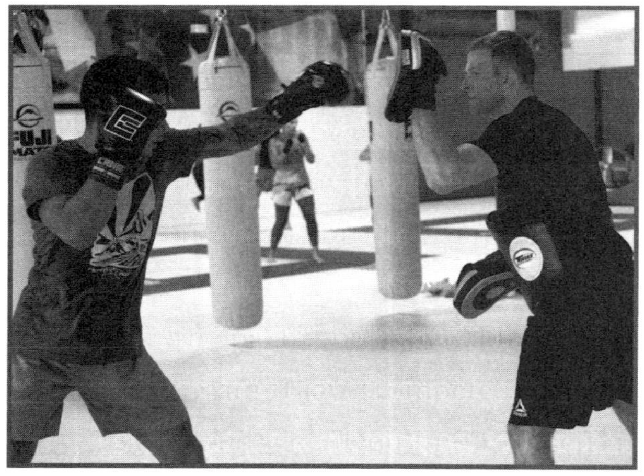

The little details make the big differences.

Seigher Brown

I dabble in photography, and years ago I was photographing a boxing event in Phoenix. I shot thousands of photos throughout the night of the four- and six- and ten-round fights. As I scrolled through the pictures later the next day, I noticed a pattern. Every single winning fighter had better technique than the losing fighter in every single picture. Every single picture! The losing fighter was slightly off-balance. Jab was too low. Right hand was extended instead of by his face. The winning fighters were on balance. Hands higher on their heads than their opponents. It wasn't a mistake; it wasn't a coincidence. They were small differences in technical ability, but compounded over four, eight, ten rounds, they made massive differences. The biggest being winning or losing.

Base balance and body control are critical to a fighter's success, just as it's critical to success in other sports (like football), especially as fatigue sets in. If you're off balance, it doesn't matter how good you are. Consider that a metaphor for life. As a coach who believes in the value of fundamentals, I try to make sure that when a fighter of mine is throwing their right hand, they're doing so while on balance, with their thumb pointed down and their chin tucked. When they pull that right hand back, our work in the gym enables them to do so in a controlled manner, without any wasted movement. I can't control what the opponent does. I can't control what the crowd does. I can't control what the judges do. But in preparation for a fight, I can make sure that your chin is down, and your hands are up and you're on balance. And generally, the fighter with the better fundamentals is going to win nine times out of ten.

A great example of this is Conor McGregor's knockout of longtime reigning Featherweight champ José Aldo at UFC 194 (2015). Aldo came out and immediately lunged in with a lead left hook. His balance was off and he overthrew the punch. Conor slid back out of the way and countered with a beautiful straight left hand that sent the champ to the canvas. At just 13 seconds into the first round, McGregor dethroned the longest-reigning Featherweight champion in UFC history.

A more recent but remarkably similar example is Sean O'Malley's victory over bantamweight champion Aljamain Sterling at UFC 292 (August 2023). In the second round O'Malley shifted his left leg backward into a southpaw stance. Aljamain lunged in the exact same way Aldo did years earlier, and the result was the exact same.

Strength and conditioning are huge factors in fights, but they usually only come into play after a few rounds have been fought and fighters begin to tire. Before fatigue plays its role, technique reigns supreme. Without technique, there's no need to worry about strength and conditioning, as rarely will the competition get to the point where it will be competitive enough to need it. This is a truism that extends far beyond the mat and applies to everything you do, whether it be your business or your life. If you are sound in your technique, you won't be the one to mess up first. And, furthermore, the greater the discrepancy between your technique and your opponent's, the less you'll need superior strength and conditioning to lead you to victory. Conversely, the closer the technical skill level, the more other factors like strength, conditioning, and psychology play a role.

Imagine you're a very good basketball player (an adult). Maybe you're a pro or maybe you played in college. Your twelve-year-old nephew challenges you to a game in the front driveway. You wouldn't even really need to try, and the final score is 11–0 in your favor. Then your sixteen-year-old nephew challenges you. You are moving a little more, and might have even broken a sweat, but you win 11–2—and the two points scored were more you not expecting her to make the shots rather than her running the paint and getting the layup. Now your younger brother challenges you to a game, and he's in his first year at college. You beat him 11–6, but he made you work and you had to actually play. You knew if you were too lazy, he'd get the rebounds. He'd score if you left him wide open. You knew you'd win, but if you took it easy, you'd definitely be hearing a jawfull at dinner. You got a good sweat going and your heart rate shot up. But now your friend challenges you to a one-on-one game. He plays on the same team as you. Everyone's watching. The score is 11–10 and it was an all-out brawl of a game. You're both sitting on the pavement dead tired and wishing you had worn better shoes! The closer you are in skill level, the more strength and conditioning come into play—so why not unlevel the playing field by being *that much better*?! Why give people a chance to outwork you?

Another, more quantitative example of this is the NFL combine. The discrepancy between technique and physical attributes is huge! If we examine the top performers throughout the NFL's combine's history, we are going to see some numbers that would make anyone feel inferior.

Prior to Xavier Worthy breaking John Ross's record in 2024, Ross held the 40-yard dash record of 4.22. Gerald Sensabaugh holds the vertical record of 46 inches and played eight years in the NFL. Stephen Paea holds the bench press record and played seven seasons in the NFL. Notice any similarities between these record holders? Before reading this, if you'd seen their names, would you recognize them? Now what about Tom Brady? Tyreek Hill? Aaron Donald? Emmitt Smith or Deion Sanders? Exactly, you don't recognize any of those record holder names, but you recognize the latter group of names as being some of the NFL's greatest ever. Do you think Tom Brady was the fastest or strongest? Not a chance. He worked hard and had the technical abilities to excel at the highest level.

See, it's not the biggest or the strongest or the fastest who tend to be the best. It helps! And you need a baseline for each. If you're TOO small or TOO weak or TOO slow, you won't be able to compete regardless of how technical you are. But once you reach a certain level of each, as the saying goes, "The Skills Pay the Bills."

PEDAGOGY: THE ART OF TEACHING . . . AND LEARNING

Teaching and discovering more effective methods of teaching and learning are some of my greatest passions. Teaching is an art, and I have practiced it in various forms for many years. My initial experience with teaching and leadership began early in my MMA career when my coach was less engaged, and I took on the task of running warm-ups—which soon moved to demonstrating techniques and leading Brazilian Jiu Jitsu and MMA classes. Then, when my

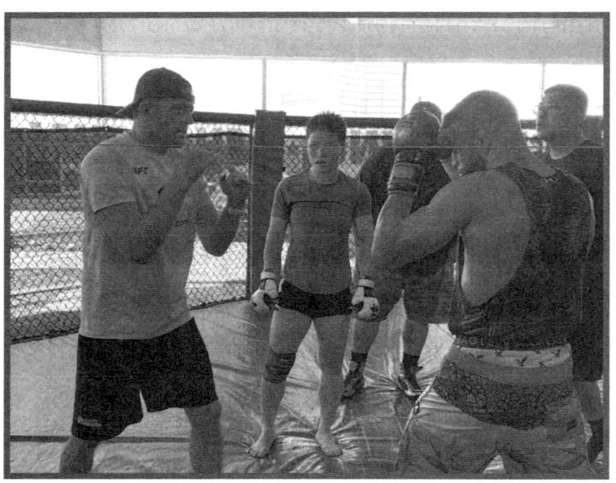

Teaching is a gift, and each student learns differently, whether because of language or learning ability. Weili Zhang is just one of the few non-English speakers I've coached over the years. *Seigher Brown*

career as a fighter was cut short by a brain aneurysm, I opened a gym and trained fighters for six years before pursuing an MFA in Creative Writing, which led to teaching English at a community college for a few years. During that time, I also conducted educational workshops for school district teachers and administrators—a friend's business—that focused on teaching through questioning methods, further deepening my understanding of pedagogy. Now, after nearly fifteen years of coaching MMA fighters since grad school, my passion for teaching continues to grow further, especially with the added curiosity and desire to educate my two young sons in sports, reading, and math.

The most exciting part of teaching is having to disseminate information to varying types of learners. On the mats I regularly engage savants and very functional humans as well as those with an IQ barely above 80. I'm coaching law school students alongside felons. English-speaking Americans and Chinese, Brazilians, Iraqis—all at the same time. The need to communicate with everyone and anyone is paramount for my athletes to actualize the success they all seek.

BEFORE WE TEACH, WE NEED TO LEARN

Of course we need to learn material before we teach it. That's a given. But how did you learn that material? What types of learning modalities did you find most effective? In high school, did you find lectures boring or thrilling? Did you learn by reading or listening? Writing things down or by photographic memory? Understanding how *we* learned material as a learner is very important as *we* educate others.

In the beginning

The learning process begins as we are pulled from our mother's womb. We see light, so we close our eyes. We feel the cold air, so we cry. Doctors and nurses pull our arms and legs and stick needles in us and probe our ears. All of these elicit a response and are stored as memories, which in turn layer upon each other every moment of our lives. Unconsciously, every single interaction with our body, with our environment, with our mind, is being catalogued. We are learning what we like and what we don't like. Pleasure and pain. A lifetime of learning has begun.

After birth, we grab things with our hands and kick our legs. We put things in our mouth, as one of the only concepts we're aware of upon birth is hunger, and fullness after eating. So, we put anything and everything into our mouths—or our mouths on anything and everything. We open our eyes. We recognize where our food comes from. We don't have a consciousness or self-awareness, but we will. We begin to experience the world. We see the world, hear the world, feel the world around us; collectively those sensational interactions create the world in which we engage. With those memories we have a recall ability (with variant capabilities), which gives us the ability to make educated predictions on what will happen next. As an infant, we cry. Our mother comes for us. We make a sound, and our father laughs. We recognize those patterns, and we repeat them. As we learn to walk, there's a combination of memory recall, muscle strength, and muscle memory. Combined we learn how to walk and crawl. It's all memory recall—at a fast pace.

Sports are no different. You have to recognize patterns quickly, which separates you from your opponent. And the more patterns an athlete recognizes faster, the more an athlete looks clairvoyant—like Nostradamus, able to see into the future. But we're not clairvoyant, we're just better at recognizing patterns faster. We see subtle weight shifts in our opponent (possibly before he even recognizes it) and we are able to move accordingly, sometimes without their awareness of the situation entirely.

We are not created equal, so choose your sport wisely

Before we get into the weeds of teaching, I do want to note that at an adult level, we must have already chosen the correct sport because that alone is one of the more crucial decisions you can make—way more important than training techniques or conditioning drills. You can only "nurture" so far before the "nature" wins.

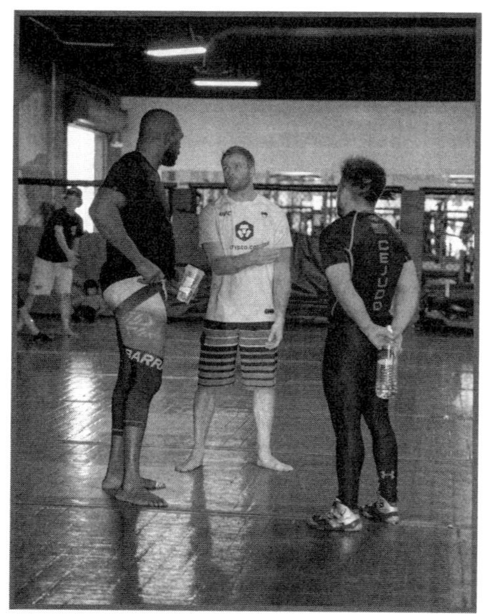

MMA is one of the few sports where athletes can have very different body types and excel. Could you imagine Henry trying to play basketball, or Jon trying to be a gymnast? *Seigher Brown*

David Epstein writes in *The Sports Gene* about the different somatotypes found in genetically African (black) humans versus those found in people from European/Scandinavian (white) countries. We generally see white swimmers and black runners at the Olympic level, and it's not a coincidence that people with longer torsos and shorter legs tend to be better swimmers, and those with longer legs and shorter torsos tend to have the advantage in running sports—especially long-distance running, where the ratio of the calf circumference to the length of leg directly correlates with marathon race times. Seeing as those with European ancestry tend to have longer torsos and shorter legs, and Africans tend to have the opposite, it makes perfect sense when we look at the Olympics and see the athletes within each event. But there's more than somatotypes to finding the "perfect" athletic endeavor for ourselves or our children.

A 5′3″ basketball player isn't going to get drafted into the NBA regardless of his 40-yard dash time or his vertical, but he may make a great gymnast or wrestler or horse jockey. A woman may be the fastest, most athletic boxer with the perfect arm reach to punch women in the face, but if she can't take a punch and gets knocked out too easily, it won't matter. If you have poor eyesight, you're not hitting home runs in MLB. Nurture versus nature is only relevant when certain genetic criteria are met, and the ubiquitous quote, "Hard work beats talent when talent doesn't work hard" is very true—to a point! So, all you raging parents out there, before you try to turn your child into the next Tom Brady or Serena Williams, look around at the family members on both parental sides of you and see if those are realistic goals. Malcom Gladwell talks about the ten-thousand-hour rule, but you can send a cheetah in the water for ten million hours, and it's not going to beat a fish in a water race.

WHAT DOES IT MEAN TO "LEARN"?

Most of what we learn at the earliest stages of our lives is through *modeling*—we observe others and then we imitate those behaviors. Listening can also be included in the modeling process—a person explains something, and then a learner attempts to act out instructions that were auditorily obtained. Modeling is a process that uses the five senses (sight and sound are the most common learning modalities and then touch; to an even lesser degree, taste and smell) to learn. As we grow older, we use more abstract forms of learning like comparing and contrasting, predicting the future and future actions based on learned knowledge and through previous experiences and teachings. And although there are numerous pedagogical approaches to teaching, for the sake of this book, many are just not realistic to bring into every facet of sports and athletics. So I want to focus on a select few that I use on a regular basis to teach my athletes.

CLASSROOM BEFORE THE FIELD

Before we dive into our physical skills training and the various phases of athletic training, we need to understand learning even more. And who better to learn from than one of the godfathers of pedagogy himself, Dr. Benjamin Bloom, the famed educational psychologist known ubiquitously in all teaching circles for his hierarchy of cognitive skills known as Bloom's Taxonomy.

If we want to learn and teach more effectively, we need to understand learning from a pedagogical point of view—from a cognitive point of view. On the next page is Bloom's Taxonomy pyramid, which breaks down the levels of learning and cognition.

Each level is arbitrarily as important as the level above or below. If you can't remember, but you can create, it won't do you very well, and vice versa. You need all levels to actualize mastery of a skill, but we generally start at the bottom and work our way upward as skills and understanding progress. The closer one gets to mastery of a skill, the more she will toggle back and forth between each level as needed.

Remember: This is the most basic level of understanding. This is your first day walking into a boxing gym and taking a few classes—a coach will tell you not to cross your feet, teach you about the stance, explain how to throw basic punches, and show you basic defenses. You will have to constantly remind yourself of the details, and although you "know" what to do, you don't really understand "why" you're doing these things or how to implement them.

BLOOM'S TAXONOMY

CREATE	**Produce new or original work** Design, assemble, construct, conjecture, develop, formulate, author, investigate
EVALUATE	**Justify a stand or decision** Appraise, argue, defend, judge, select, support, value, critique, weigh
ANALYZE	**Draw connections among ideas** Differentiate, organize, relate, compare, contrast, distinguish, examine, experiment, question, test
APPLY	**Use information in new situations** Execute, implement, solve, use, demonstrate, interpret, operate, schedule, sketch
UNDERSTAND	**Explain ideas or concepts** Classify, describe, discuss, explain, identify, locate, recognize, report, select, translate
REMEMBER	**Recall fact and basic concepts** Define, duplicate, list, memorize, repeat, state

In standard education, the remember section would be reading a text out loud or memorizing a chart. It doesn't mean you understand any of it, but you can state it and start the memorization process.

Understand: Now you understand your basic punch combinations and defenses and why you don't cross your feet while stepping to your left or right. You understand how to slip a punch and why you want your weight on this foot or that foot depending on what punch you're throwing. This level doesn't mean you can actually beat anyone up in sparring, but you understand certain functions, and you can start to have fun—even if you're the one taking the beating, as opposed to giving one.

In standard education, this would mean you're not only reading the text, but you're able to explain it as well. You're not just memorizing equations, but you're walking through them step-by-step.

Apply: This is the big learning phase in a sport. Most athletes will spend a lot of time in this phase, as this is where you're going to get a lot of minutes in the ring, or on a field, learning your craft. Now, you're sparring and getting rounds in again and again. Little by little you begin to hone your skills. This is a long phase and encompasses everything from "just getting good enough to spar" to "he's getting really good." Your jab goes from loose and wide to straight and crisp. Your balance is better. Eventually, you begin to become one of the better fighters in your skill level (controlled for size, weight, time in sport).

In standard education, you're now able to compute those same math questions without the help of a step-by-step guide. At first, you get more wrong than right but, eventually, you begin to get more and more correct, and you are able to complete them in a more timely manner.

Analyze: You've gotten past the point of basic understanding and now you're going to start to add your own spin on things. Up until this point, you've probably heavily relied on your instructors to teach you your techniques, but now you're seeing techniques while watching fights or other training videos, and you're adding those techniques to your arsenal. You're now blending your boxing with your kicks, your wrestling with your strikes. You're able to distinguish between a traditional Thai style kickboxer and a Dutch style kickboxer—and you're taking pieces of each and adding them into your own arsenal. Also, this is when you start to make moves "your own." You change up details just a bit from how you were taught to better suit your own game. You begin to do things differently—not in a bad way or a way that is far from your own technical level, but you make that technical level specific to you.

In standard education, this would be when you're able to compare and contrast when you're reading an essay in the classroom. You're already good enough to analyze the essay on an individual basis, but now you're able to take another topic and find similarities in an otherwise dissimilar topic/situation and also find differences between two seemingly similar topics/situations.

Evaluate: Now you're confident. You've been training a long time, and you not only know what you know, but you now understand what others know and if the techniques are right or wrong for a given situation. You have your own voice. You have your own style now. Someone shows you a technique and you can say, "No, I don't like that" or "I do that this way" or even "I do like that technique and here's why or how I'd use it" (which might be different than how you were shown to use it). While sparring, people know what you are going to do, but you're still able to implement your game plan regardless. You trust your coach, but he also trusts you and your judgment to make calls on the fly.

In traditional education, you are now able to critique an argument. You are knowledgeable enough to say, "No, I don't agree with that statement/point of view and here's why." Not only do you argue against a certain point of view, but you have logic and facts that can back it up. Your arguments are compelling.

Create: This is Bloom's final, and highest, form of pedagogy—the ability to create something new. As a fighter, you may be at the highest level where you're creating new movements, new combinations. This is where Anthony Pettis found his jump-off-the-cage kicks. This is where Imanari found out you could roll into a leg lock from a standing position. You've created something new—whether it's a single move or an entire system. People begin to copy your moves and make their own spin on them (this person is using part of the "analyze" phase). When you reach this level of competency, you might not even be fighting anymore. You may not even reach this level until well into your coaching years.

In traditional education, this is where scholarly research comes in. This is where new information comes from. New inventions. New medicines. This is even above a traditional high school teacher's level of understanding, and goes into the PhD level of understanding.

That's where Bloom ends, but I have another stage, and this is the stage athletes need to understand and engage in. There isn't a single physical attribute that will predict athletic success as much as this next stage.

Predict: From the outside, great athletes seem to be superhuman—they look faster than everybody else, or stronger, or never miss a free throw due to their homing device. In reality, though, speed and strength and homing devices are not what separate good athletes from average athletes or great athletes from the good ones. The elite athletes do possess a superpower, though. But they share more in common with Nostradamus than the physical specimen likely standing next to him in the training room.

What separates the elite athletes from the rest is their ability to tell the future . . . well, that's a little hyperbolic, but they can do a damn good job of predicting it—and they do so based on pattern recognition, not psychic powers.

FIVE STAGES OF ATHLETIC LEARNING: STATIC DRILLING, VARIANT DRILLING, LIGHT LIVE DRILLING, LIVE DRILLING, AND CHESS VISUALIZATION

Bloom's Taxonomy of cognitive skills broke down the levels of learning used in a classroom. On the following pages, I have translated those into how I break down athletic training, as many blend into one, as well as added some variation. Understanding Bloom's Taxonomy is one thing, but being able to take that and translate it into usable, athletic terms is what we're here for. You will see numerous similarities. This section, at first, may seem redundant, but read deeper and you'll see Bloom's stages don't match up perfectly with athletics. Some stages are blended together, while others are added. And classroom theory doesn't always translate to real-world application so smoothly.

Static drilling

The first stage of athletic learning is static drilling. There are two sublevels to static drilling: unconscious static and conscious static. Unconscious is, most commonly, the most basic form of modeling that you can find. You will circle back to this level at the elite level, but now, as a beginner, this stage is more of Simon Says than anything you have a real understanding of. Simon tells you to raise your hand; you raise your hand. He says to jump; you jump. You don't know why. You just do as you're told. You're brand new to a sport—day one in tennis. You learn to hold the racket. You learn how to stand. Eventually you learn how to swing your new racket. Everything feels foreign. The stance is hard to maintain. Your back hurts. The racket keeps tilting inward. You aren't following through on your strokes.

Your tennis pro comes along and tells you (verbally) to turn your racket out and swing again. You do so again and again. He may pantomime the move. He gets in his stance and gives you some details. Some talking points. He swings and swings. You watch. Then you repeat again and again. Either he is hitting balls directly in an area for you to hit with minimal movement or you are swinging at air. There is zero resistance in your line of movement. You can freely drill the move again and again with zero variance.

In fighting, this might be shadowboxing or bag work or partner drills. There is a very specific task. You perform numerous repetitions, and then you move on to a new task, or even add onto that task and create a chain of tasks. First, you throw twenty-five jabs. Then you throw twenty-five jab-cross combinations. Then you add on and after the jab-cross, you slip a punch and throw a hook.

Shooting baskets would be another example of static drilling. You stand at a free throw line and shoot a basket. Then you move and shoot a three-pointer. You move again, and work a fadeaway jumper. You can shoot a million times from a million different points on the court in a million different manners, but if you're the only one on the court, you don't have a variant. A variant is something that changes. In sports, a variant is your opponent or training partner or terrain change.

Static drilling is the first level of learning anything. You don't even know where you're supposed to go, or stand, or even how to stand or how to swing. This is the foundation. When most people think of learning, this is what comes to mind. But static drilling is important in another phase of training, and usually forgotten once athletes get the nuts and bolts of a sport, as so many mediocre athletes just want to "play" or "go live" and, oftentimes, want to push too hard and get a "workout." Being good at a sport is more akin to computer coding or surgery than "getting a good workout" though, and that's what a lot of mediocre athletes don't understand. You wouldn't want the fastest surgeon, would you? He comes in, chops you up, and moves on to the next—getting as many surgeries in as he can. You want someone who, when she trained to be a surgeon, took her time and worked meticulously at perfecting the surgical process. Eventually, of course, the speed will increase, but quality over quantity reigns supreme in surgery, and athletics. This second form of static drilling comes in the form of conscious static drilling. This is what separates the good from the exceptional and the exceptional from the true greats of a sport.

We'll come full circle and talk more about conscious static drilling at the end of our learning phase.

Variant drilling

Static drilling is a great introduction into sport, or anything, but it's not really real. Standing in a completely controlled environment performing a technique in a vacuum is great as a learning tool, but it won't prepare you for actual competition.

A great book to read on the mind and how it works and processes variant and invariant patterns is Jeff Hawkins' *On Intelligence.* Hawkins was the inventor of the PalmPilot, a personal assistant device that was one of the early adopters of very basic artificial intelligence (but we'll use that term very loosely here, as it's completely different from the AI we know today). In the book, he details human brain function and learning processes as opposed to how computers function. We've heard so often that the human brain is more powerful than the world's most powerful supercomputer that many of us actually believe it. We've been told we only use 10 percent of our brain, and if we used 100 percent, we'd have superpowers. But those two things, as Hawkins says, are very untrue. To address the latter first—yes, we may only use 10 percent of our brain . . . but that's at a time. Most of our day-to-day functions don't require all our brain power. Our brain may use the medulla oblongata to regulate our heart or cough or sneeze, but when we're working through Descartes or processing a breakup with a lover, the frontal lobe is active. Each part of the brain is responsible for different human functions, so why would it need to be active at the same time? That would be like turning all of the lights on in your house. It would be a complete waste of electricity. But walking in a dark room, turning the light on while you're inside, and then turning the light off when you leave makes way more sense. We only need light in the room if we're in the room. We only need each part of the brain turned on when we're using that part of the brain. And to the former, the brain is NOT more powerful than a supercomputer by any stretch of the imagination, but it is significantly more efficient than one. See, the brain takes shortcuts. After it learns a process, it doesn't have to relearn/reprocess that information every single time. It makes note of the process and picks up where you left off last time. The brain has an autosave function similar to your word processing software on your computer—you're not rewriting the story every single time you want to add a chapter. You save the chapter and start from where you left off. The brain is also very efficient with its physical makeup. It is layered in a series of folds, which makes it much easier for one part of the brain to make connections with other parts of the brain if needed. Well, why is this important? Variability, that's why. Humans have it, computers don't (really), and it is huge in the sports learning world, whether you know it or not.

Variability is exactly as it sounds, a variant of something. Not something completely new, but only slightly so. If you have a red and a blue marble, they aren't different things. They are just different colors. A variant of one another. Hawkins uses the example in *On Intelligence* of a robot moving from point A to point B. Early robot machines could process that task. Move from this part of a room to that part of a room, pick up an object, and then bring it back to the starting point. But if marbles or cut-up cardboard or other obstructions were placed in its line of movement, it couldn't process the task. It looked at the obstruction as a separate task, and it wasn't programmed to perform that task. Humans, without reprogramming, can make observations about a variant without as much thought.

When a fighter is throwing his rear hand at an opponent, we generally call that a “cross” or “overhand.” The main difference between the two is the arch in which the punch is thrown. A cross tends to leave the body in a straight manner, whereas an overhand is thrown more with an arc like a baseball or football—for lack of a better description: Cross equals straight; overhand equals arc. But for this explanation, we’re going to lump them together. If an opponent throws a “straight” with a little bit of an arc, the brain would still process that as a “right hand” (if in an orthodox stance) and if more arc was added, it would be the same. And more arc? Well, the same. The same goes for a jab. If the thumb is up, it’s a jab. Turn the thumb down a bit, and it’s a jab. Turn the thumb down farther, well, it’s still a jab. Our human brains are capable of recognizing the patterns between two seemingly different punches and categorizing them together. Now, if a jab was thrown with a left hand and then a hook was thrown afterward, even though they are thrown with the same hand/arm, our brain recognizes two distinctly different punches are coming at us. We need to recognize the similarities between things and categorize them appropriately.

By adding variants, we add marbles to our path . . . but we find a way around them on our own. If you were playing tennis, your coach would now place balls slightly in front of you as you practice your backhand, forcing you to adjust your position forward. Next, he’d place the ball a bit to your right, and then maybe barely out of your reach, so you’d fail to return the ball. All of which forced you to make adjustments and learn from each (especially the failure!), but you’re still confined to hitting with just the backhand stroke. You’re not “playing live” as there are still constraints placed upon the drilling exercise to work a specific task. Variant drilling still focuses on a specific technical drill, but the variants inject a bit of free thinking into the mix.

Variant drilling introduces success and failure into technical components of a sport that allow for microadjustments with every repetition of the movement. The real benefit to variant drilling is that the feedback loop (whether something works or not) is immediate (either something works or it doesn't) and then an athlete gets to try another option—WITHOUT BEING COACHED. And that's a huge deal. Just like small children not asking for help with getting their scooter over a pothole, we need athletes to figure out problems as well. Resiliency is key, as is problem-solving. Having a coach give us all the answers is akin to cheating on the math test. For me, I never want the answer told to me. I want to figure it out on my own like a riddle or magic trick. The joy comes from the problem-solving and doing the work, not the answer. I doubt you'd gloat after cheating on a test and receiving an A. Either cheat in silence, or study and EARN the A, but being proud of a fake grade is as silly to me as wanting the answer told to me while wrestling or hitting a tennis ball—of course, at the infancy stage of a sport, you ask questions and need answers, but you're past that now. Act like it! You'll also learn more from your failures than you will from your successes. If you fail twenty-five times at a task, you know exactly what not to do in the future, and as new scenarios present themselves, whether in practice or live competition, the knowledge of that failed movement will guide you to another alternative when in need of an impromptu solution.

Light live training

Light live drilling is a great, fun way to acclimate athletes to live play. Light sparring (for fighting) or noncompetitive tennis matches are a fun way to try to win, but not at all costs. As a boxer, you don't care if you're getting hit with a jab five hundred times a round, as you're trying to work an overhand right into the mix. Winning the round isn't important. The win comes by achieving a specific micro goal within that round. In this scenario, landing an overhand right. Too often, gym heroes try to win every round and every moment of every practice, even at the expense of getting better and improving. Their ego won't allow them to think someone else won, even if they are trying a new move. Light live is how beginners become comfortable getting from the drilling stage to the live stage. This stage is where so much athletic growth comes from. Sometimes you will actually try to win the round. Other times you'll intentionally place yourself at a disadvantage and try to dig yourself out of the hole—dig yourself out of the intentional constraint. The constraint may be a specific punch you're trying to land (offensive constraint) or by using limiting constraints—taking away athletic weapons, such as only using your backhand in tennis or by strictly using a jab in boxing. "Playing" light allows for free play and free thought, without the worry of being hurt by a sparring partner (ensure you and your training partner are on the same page with the intensity level). It allows for constant adjustments and feedback, just as variant drilling allows, but this is live play, so athletes can work a realistic scenario.

Live training

We're going! Live training is putting the pads on, strapping up the football helmet, going eleven on eleven, and trying to win. Live training is playing a full quarter or half or game of basketball—five on five and we're trying to win. Fighters, this is sparring and we're going as hard as we can to simulate a real fight—as hard as we can without hurting each other. Live training is needed to see what you can perform when it matters. Live training is the closest thing to actual competition you can get. It's a critical component.

At our gym, Fight Ready MMA, we spar hard on Tuesdays and Fridays. Those with a fight scheduled will perform their sparring rounds in the cage. A list is formulated and each fighter will have sparring partners listed for one to five rounds, depending on the details of the upcoming fight. While cage rounds are going on, other fighters are sparring out in the open, on the mats. The sparring is much more intense than light live rounds, but nowhere near what's going on in the cage.

When a fighter first comes into the gym and has his first cage round, there's almost always panic in his face. Both before going in, and definitely when coming out. If sparring outside, he can spar for three or five or eight rounds of five minutes each. Whatever. But during cage rounds, he is dead tired midway through one round or, if he's lucky, two rounds. But why? It's the "realness" of the situation. Scores of people may be huddled up around the cage, spectating. There's an opponent across the cage from you who's going to try to beat you up. On the outside, it doesn't matter if you get hit or land a takedown. Inside the cage it does. These are your rounds, and you need to prove to yourself you can win them when it matters. The punches come hard. People need stitches after having their eyes ripped open from an errant elbow or knee. Some get knocked out. It's not malice or carnage we're seeking, but we have to test ourselves in a situation where we can really see if what we're practicing will work. Maybe the worst part, though—adrenaline. Taming the adrenaline is huge, and it's omnipresent during competition, and it's the greatest tool and the greatest detriment all at once. It's how you balance it that matters.

I always tell people that we don't really know who the best boxer or basketball player in the world is. That guy's in the gym beating the brakes off world champions somewhere. Or draining threes on Jordan or Lebron in a practice room. We only see who the best is when millions of people are watching—who the best is when things matter. And there's a big difference in who the best is in the practice room and who the best is on Monday Night Football. We must train as hard as we can every once in a while, to try to simulate that adrenaline. To simulate live play. And the amazing catches in practice and head movement and three-sixty fadeaway jump shots you hit in the practice gym mean nothing unless you can hit them when a championship is on the line.

Chess visualization

Most of us are familiar with chess—the sophisticated board game with the goal of capturing an opponent's king. Each separate piece has different rules as to the pattern in which it's allowed to move throughout the board. The complex rule structure for each piece makes it difficult to see which pieces of your own might be in danger of being captured. To win, you'll need to think multiple moves ahead, but it isn't a linear game like Connect 4. In Connect 4, toward the end of the game, you can count out which color would go in each slot. Red. Blue. Red. Blue. Darn. I Lose. With chess, there's a four-dimensional component—you need to have the ability to see many moves ahead but, remember, each piece can move differently than each other piece, and there may be numerous pieces (of both yours and your opponent's), which may create a myriad of options. It's a Choose Your Own Adventure book, but instead of adding, or even multiplying, numbers, we're dealing with exponents—scores of options, hundreds of options. Maybe more. And one of the greatest differentiators that separates varying levels of chess players (and the level they play at) is the ability to plan the game out in their head, which, in part, includes the ability to visualize more gameplay moves ahead than their opponent.

The ability to visualize the next move, and then the potential counterattack (and then the next attack-counter-attack-counter etc.) is crucial to learning.

I'll admit, I like chess, and have played casually throughout my life, but I never really took to it for numerous reasons. Somehow, I took this "visualizing each move and playing the game out in my head" style of learning into martial arts. But there's an additional component that is inserted into our visualization for sports. In chess, we're visualizing other objects and mapping out a series of possible future attacks for our own pieces as well as our opponent's possible counterattacks. We're sequencing abstractly—because we are not visualizing our self. With our athletic endeavors, the pieces we're visualizing are our own body parts, as well as those of our opponents. Fortunately for us, there's a mind-body connection activated during visualization that has more benefits than we could dream of. How many times have you been daydreaming of a physical activity only to have your arm twitch, or your leg lurch? That's not a coincidence, and there's a lot of science backing the mind-body connection in sports.

In a study with 120 student participants, Peynircioğlu, Thompson, and Tanielian tested basketball free throw shooting before and after various types of visual imagery. Those assigned to imagery "interventions" demonstrated a 7.4% improvement in free throw shooting compared to matched control groups who received no mental training. Another experiment by Arsiwi and colleagues tested video-based visualization with 24 male athletes and documented a statistically significant increase: free throw scores rose from a mean of 6.25 before training to 8.54 after just four weeks, showing a 37% improvement over baseline. At the elite level of basketball, Guillot et al. showed that ten high-level basketball athletes practicing static motor imagery improved their shooting accuracy by 44%.

As an early grappler on my MMA journey, I adopted the chess visualization routine. I've grappled and trained some sort of combative sport most of my life, so I can visualize movements and "feel" them in a manner consistent with actual physical touch. I assume most athletes can visualize an athletic movement and create a visceral experience with it after a certain baseline of skill has been met as well.

In the evenings, after training, I'd go home and sit on my couch and recap the day's training. I'd revisit random moments of my training—the good, the bad, and the confusing—with a specific focus on problems I couldn't solve during the training itself. I hate losing, but I love riddles, so I'd try to solve the riddles of the day. One day I was submitted in an arm bar. Immediately after being submitted, I did what I always do when I lose—I put myself back in the exact same position/scenario. I wanted to see what I did wrong. Of course, I got submitted again. "Okay, got it. This is what he's doing," I thought. Instead of avoiding the situation altogether, I threw myself into the same position. Got submitted. Then I put my arm near the same position, but not quite as deep. I got submitted. I tend to do that when I lose. I want to re-create the scenario as much as possible, so I understand every single possible outcome when I encounter it again. But the problem is . . . time (and willing partners). There's not enough time in a round for me to get as many do-overs as I need to figure out the "chess problem." And rarely is there a partner who is going to keep doing the same crazy thing as many times as I need to get to the comfort level that I want to be at. So, I sit on my couch and visualize being submitted. "I put my arm here, and lost, so what if I did this instead?" I visualize the moment. I can feel my opponent's legs and hips and where my balance is. "He'd then do this or that." *I lose.* In my visualized sequence, I lost. I play it out again. I move my arm. He counters. I recounter. I play out every sequence again and again. I lose. Again and again, my brain processes the outcomes and spits out losses after losses. But, even with every loss, I get better. I already know what those losses feel like in the real world, as I felt them in my focused session of visualization—preventing real losses the next time I find myself in that position in the gym. And, eventually, I find my win. I reprocess it a few times, and it checks out. The next day I'll go into the gym and try it out in real life. And the good news: It almost always works out the way it played out in my head!

I learned and improved while sitting on my couch.

Static drilling (conscious)

It's time to circle back. I talked about unconscious drilling earlier—the Simon Says version of learning. But now you know what you're doing. You know your sport. You've traveled through the different training stages and you're getting better—or maybe you're already great. But that's not enough. Good isn't enough. Hell, great isn't enough. And even if it is "enough" you want to get better still. You want to perfect what you know and create what hasn't been before. This is where conscious drilling comes into play.

You're swinging a tennis racket. You're already good, and you know how to swing. You know how to play. You know the rules of tennis. You KNOW tennis. There's a rule in writing—you need to know the rules, and then you can break the rules. It's time to break the rules . . . sort of. And now, since you know the rules of tennis, or basketball, or fighting, it's time to break them, or at least break your own rules and patterns.

On the court, you find yourself swinging for lower balls with your arm outstretched and you want to change that. So you go back to your Simon Says reps. You drill what you've been taught. But then you change it on your own. You play with the angle. Instead of reaching out with your arm, you bend at the waist—it feels foreign, but you do it again. You then bend your legs. Again, you play with the angle of the arm and racket. You drill again and again and again—each time you make mental notes. You find a new solution to how you hit that same type of ball and you drill it a hundred times. Each repetition has its own mental tag. You're making the adjustments and perfecting them again and again. You don't need a partner (but you can certainly do this with partners too), and it's all making sense.

This same scenario could be on a basketball court. You watch the tape of a game, and your game winning three-pointer was blocked. You notice the arc of the ball and the angle of your wrist. You practice with different release techniques for days and weeks and months to see if a new angle will provide you with the extra inch clearance you need when you face that team again next year.

This last stage of learning is when the beautiful moments of sports are made. These are how the Aaron Rodgerses hit that no-look pass and the Odell Beckham Jr.s pull in that uncatchable ball with one hand. Conscious drilling is what breeds greatness. The best part about this phase, though, is that it can be incorporated anywhere throughout the athletic ladder—but most lose sight of it during the process and can't take a step backward long enough to climb ten steps higher.

Tim Tebow was a Heisman Trophy winner in college and was selected twenty-fifth overall in the 2010 NFL draft. He was supposed to be a franchise quarterback—he was supposed to be a guy who stayed in the league for years. He was "Him." Until he wasn't. He played for the Denver Broncos for two years and was then traded to the NY Jets. Afterward, he spent time with the Patriots, Eagles, and then Jaguars before he finally called it quits on his NFL career. We could spend hours analyzing why Tebow wasn't a successful quarterback, but a few analysts credit his slow release time as being one of the main culprits. See, quarterbacks need to get the ball out fast. Really fast—as the average release time for a top-tier quarterback is approximately 450 milliseconds. Tebow had an average release time of nearly 557 milliseconds. One possible reason for this was his tendency to drop his hand toward his hip during his windup, causing a longer overall delay in release. Something so subtle, and minuscule to the layman, is the difference in staying in the NFL or not. Understanding such subtleties, and taking the time to improve them—consciously—could mean the difference between being a successful NFL quarterback and going home.

LEARNING IN ACTION

You now know numerous different modalities to learn during different stages, so let's give you the ability to put this into real-world practice and actually improve, as opposed to understanding some vague conceptual theory that doesn't translate into athletic improvement

1. **Practice the basics every day.** Warm up with them (shadowbox, bag work). Any skill that isn't practiced begins to fade. People believe they can outgrow fundamentals, and that's not true. If your coach doesn't systemize a warm-up incorporating fundamentals at the beginning of each practice session, show up early and work for twenty minutes on your own. Set a time for three-minute rounds and spend a round with dribbling to get your hand-eye coordination synced. Then a round on dribbling and cutting left and right. A round on free throw shooting. A round on fadeaways. Whatever you know you need to practice. And do it every day!

2. **Slow down.** Consciously train. Have training goals. They could be something simple like keeping your left hand up when you throw a punch or on the macro level of defending takedowns better (which is probably a months-long goal), but stick with it, and be conscious of it while training. Don't just coast throughout your training. Stop trying to win during practice. Some days you just try to win. Other days you need to work on something specific. It could be something technical, cardio, etc., but try to just get better at that one thing, then you have these mini wins and losses and it helps your overall mental state too—you can't redline your body or mind every day. This "slower brain" training can be done while in a variable drilling stage, or during light live training. Work toward something specific; otherwise you're just doing busywork.

3. **Become an expert at your sport.** Watch film. You'll learn so much from watching others do it. And you can learn in the classroom just as you do on the field or in the cage—football players watch an insane amount of film. Whatever sport you're engaged in, there's film. Watch religiously. Pick up on good and bad tendencies. Compare how you move and train with how the pros

are moving, and then emulate them. Re-create their movements. Don't try to copy them. Copies are never great, but drill their movements and then make them your own.

4. **Visualize.** You can only practice so many hours a day. There's only so much the body can handle on a physical level before diminishing returns set in. And there's only so many practice partners willing to engage your obsession. Spending time visualizing your sport will absolutely improve your performance. Visualize patterns. Visualize movements. Try to create riddles and solve them within your sport. You will improve!

5. **Coach.** The saying, "If you really want to know, teach," is as true as it gets. Teaching a skill requires you to look at things from a different angle. To look at things from someone else's point of view. You may try to explain the skill the way you learned it, and someone's looking back at you like a deer in the headlights. They don't get it. So, you'll have to explain from a different angle. Your understanding of the task will become multidirectional. While teaching, you'll also find yourself parroting what coaches/teachers have said to you, and you'll have your own "aha" moment, and those instructions will now make more sense than ever before. Your understanding of whatever you're teaching will become infinitely stronger from teaching.

"I CAN TEACH YOU HOW TO PUNCH AND KICK BUT I CAN'T TEACH YOU HOW TO FIGHT."

When we talk about technique, we have to break down that word. What are the technical aspects of a quarterback in football? Is it how he throws the ball? Or is it how he reads the field? Those are both technical components of being an adept quarterback, but one is a "mechanical" technique, whereas the other is an "IQ" technique.

ONE SIZE DOES NOT FIT ALL

One of the first things coaches should learn when dealing with any athlete is "don't coach athletes to perform like other athletes." Stop trying to teach Muhammad Ali–style footwork. Stop trying to teach people to catch like Odell Beckham Jr. To hit a tennis ball like Roger Federer. And athletes, run from a coach who tries to teach you to fight/perform like others, especially like her/him (the coach)—especially if you see the rounds on social media—or who tries to teach you too much theory and "if this, then that" type of stuff. The best coaches teach the fundamentals. And there's always a lot of wiggle room in every sport of what's right and wrong versus what is preferential to an individual athlete, but there are certain foundational truths that must be met. For boxing, you need to be on balance at all times. Have proper footwork. Don't overreach on your punches. Return your punches to a balanced stance. And keep your head offline and moving. There are other "rules" as well, but you get the point. After those basic techniques/foundations are met, it's not up to me as a coach to teach you how to move or really even what combos to throw. Those are things that you, as an athlete, must figure out! I'm not going to show a 5′2″ male fighter who weighs 200 lb. how to fight like a 6′ girl who weighs 130 lb. Once you start to move a certain way and show an affinity toward a movement or combination, then we'll guide you through options and drills to help accentuate those movements, but again, I can't teach that. And I certainly can't do anything about it mid-fight. But what I can do as a coach is make sure that when you're working with me, your hands are up, you're on balance, you're exiting your combinations safely, etc. If we could mimic other people's play and style and movements, we'd all be Canelo or Tom Brady, but those idiosyncrasies are unique to the individual. There is only so much you can learn from others; at some point you need to find your own style.

Imagine you enroll in an art program and study all of the paintings of times past. You learn the impressionist style of Monet, the expressionist style of Van Gogh, or the surrealism of Salvador Dalí—the brushstrokes, the color structures, the themes. You spend years learning and copying them. Then you graduate. Are you an artist? Does understanding what other people painted make you an artist? You studied how they painted. You copied the paintings. You can pick them all out of a lineup.

After graduation, you don't know what to paint, so you copy one of the greats. Maybe you have your own subject—a modern woman instead of a bearded man—would that sell? Would anyone want it? Even so, does copying a painting, or even a style, make you an artist? After graduating school, you aren't an artist. You just have the tools and the knowledge to become an artist. At best, you're prepared to be a critic, but studying others doesn't make you great by any means. But now it's time to experiment and create. To broaden and explore. Now it's time to put paint on canvas. And at first, those paintings are going to die in the garbage. They're not worthy of eyes or praise. They are reps. Just like reps swinging a tennis racket or baseball bat or throwing a punch. And they are probably bad reps. You'll want them in the trash. But little by little, those reps improve, they become sharper, more vibrant, they create their own style and scream of a uniqueness perfectly you. Graduating from art school doesn't make you an artist any more than having someone show you how to punch or what combos to throw makes you a fighter.

I've seen so many people hit a bag and rapid-fire away on focus mitts on Instagram. They look like Floyd Mayweather, but then they spar, they get in the ring or cage, and whither. Wilt. Embarrass themselves in front of everyone. Because I can't turn anyone into a fighter. I can only teach them to punch and kick. Your wide receiver coach can't turn you into a football player. He can give you the tools to break off on a route. He can teach you to get close before you break left or right. He can feed you hundreds of throws to get the reps. He can show you film of what others have done. But when the game is on, and there's a cornerback pushing you and yelling and it's raining and there's thousands of people in the stands, nobody can help you. You can't fake that.

LESS MAY BE MORE

We tend to look for answers when we lose or encounter difficulty. Generally, those answers are some form of "add this" to your regimen. Try this new combination. Try this new move. More. More. More. And "more" may very well be the answer to a lot of athletic roadblocks. But more tends to work better at the macro level.

NFL play calling and schemes have gotten significantly more advanced over the last decade. We're seeing more motion than we've seen in times past. We're seeing trick plays—flea flickers, reversals, and underhanded pitches—all considered juvenile and high schoolish by traditional NFL coaches. In MMA, we're seeing more feints and movement than ever before too. Fighters aren't necessarily trying to throw more or wrestle more, but they're faking both a lot more. Showing a move—trying to keep their opponents guessing. Smoke and mirrors. We need smoke screens in athletics. Winning and losing can very often come down to a fake punt or a trick shot. But those are outliers. You can only rely on smoke and mirrors so many times before opponents become savvy to the tricks. Often, you just need substance. You just need less.

The jack-of-all-trades is a master of none, and sometimes we need to cut out and refine. Cael Sanderson is considered the greatest collegiate wrestler of all time. He finished his NCAA career undefeated with a record of 159–0, and he is the only wrestler to ever go undefeated throughout his entire collegiate career. He won four national titles, and then went on to win gold at the 2004 Athens Olympics. His "move" was an ankle pick. Everyone knew it was coming; few could stop it. Of course he knew a million other moves, but he relied on one time and time again.

ONE LAST THING BEFORE WE GO

I fear not the man who has practiced 10,000 kicks once, but I fear the man who has practiced one kick 10,000 times.

—Bruce Lee

But Cael wasn't just a master of one move, he was special, and there's something to note about special people. Prior to his Olympic run, Cael wrestled at Iowa State under coach Bobby Douglas. He wasn't alone, though, and he certainly wasn't the only good high school wrestler in the room. He wasn't even the only good collegiate wrestler in the room, either. But there was something different about him than every other wrestler in that room, and in the history of the sport, for that matter. But what? Was he the most athletic wrestler ever? Probably not. He most likely wasn't even the most athletic guy in his wrestling room at Iowa. Did he get special treatment or coaching? Probably not. He was in a top Division I wrestling program in the nation—a lot of talented wrestlers received top-notch coaching from the talented staff of coaches. Again, then, what set him apart? Every other athlete in his high school wrestling room and college room was probably similar in athleticism, coaching, access to techniques.

What is it that set Cael Sanderson apart from the rest of the wrestlers? What is it that separates the elites from the good, and the good from the mediocre? Why didn't that high school all-star make it at the junior college level? Why didn't the girl on the freshman volleyball team, who seemed to be as good as everyone else, if not better, make it onto the Olympic team? What makes a Michael Jordan or a Lebron James or a Floyd Mayweather THAT much better than the rest of us? How do they achieve so much success? At what point do the elites separate from the pack and become these phenomenal players, and how?

I'm assuming you want the answer here, but the truth is, I don't have one for you. If you ask the greats what the difference is between them and the second best, they would probably say, "I just wanted it more than everyone else." I asked Henry Cejudo (two-division UFC champion and Olympic Gold medalist) what made him different? What made him special? He replied, "I just hate to lose. I hate losing so much more than I like winning. I hate losing."

A lot of really successful people can't articulate why they are successful—why they are great. They "just hate losing" or "wanted to be the best." And that was their drive. To some, that might mean working harder. To others, it means working smarter. And yet, to others, maybe it's watching film or adding cartwheels to a workout. My point is, you need to find out how you can separate yourself from the other high-level athletes around you. If there was a recipe on Pinterest on how to be the best ever, we'd all be cooking that meal—but even then, if we all had the secret, and we all executed that secret to a T, wouldn't we all be the same? Someone would have to break free and separate themself from the pack—but how? That's the great riddle.

So train. Play. Compete. And then repeat the process again and again and again. And when you find yourself understanding, pay closer attention. When you find yourself winning, work harder. When you find yourself losing, work twice as hard. If you find yourself losing a lot, analyze your situation. Analyze your training. Analyze your effort. You may need a change . . . or you may be doing every single thing perfectly, and you just need more time.

4

PREPARATION LEADS TO SUCCESS

There's no such thing as being too prepared. The fighter who studies his or her opponent's tendencies, visualizes every potential scenario, puts in all the mental and physical reps required, and focuses his or her attention squarely on the task at hand will not deviate from the fight plan if and when adversity strikes and will instead be able to calmly execute with precision and confidence. The countless repetitions in the gym, in the film room, and in moments of quiet contemplation enable fighters to act instinctually and rely on muscle memory instead of making risky, split-second calculations. Preparation becomes addictive once you see how powerful it is. The more work you put in, the more the fight slows down.

NOSTRADAMUS: ALWAYS KNOWS THE FUTURE

Remember the first time you played *Super Mario Bros.*? Doesn't matter which one or on which console. You barely made it 5 percent into the level, and you fell down a hole, or the little toothed mushroom, Goomba, got you. You played again and got a little farther this time—not because you were any better, but because you knew where the hole was and which beast was going to come next.

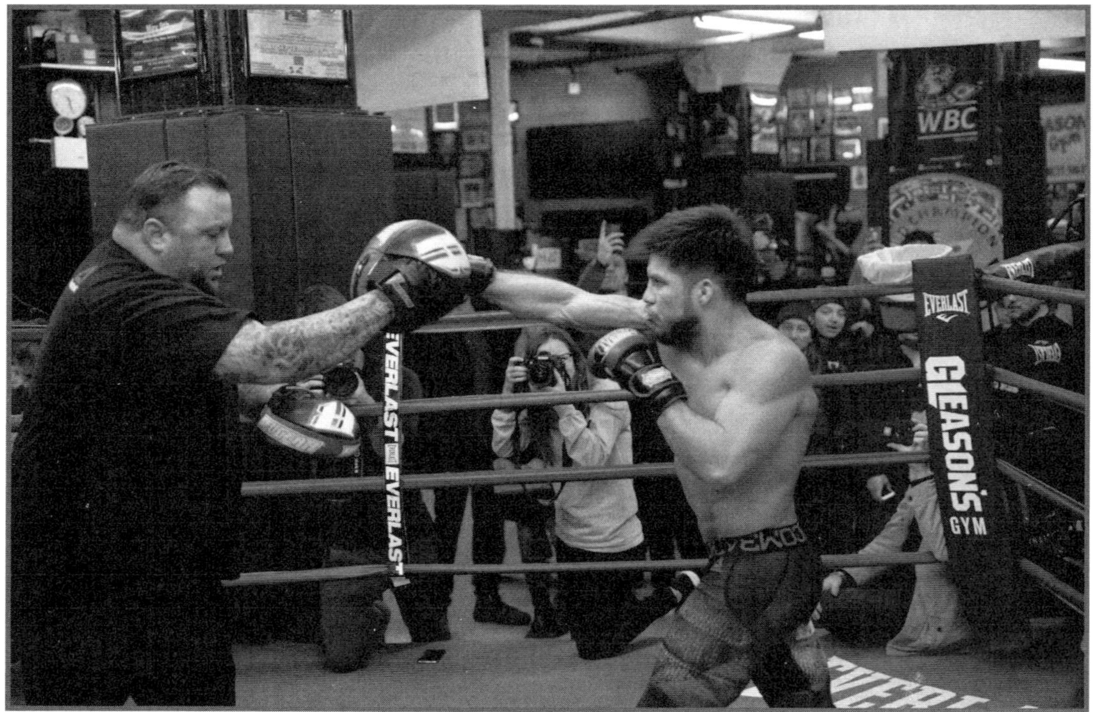

Henry works out at the famed Gleason's gym in Brooklyn before his fight with TJ Dillashaw.
Seigher Brown

Little by little you played the level again and again, and you passed it. At some point, you probably played that level so well you could fly through it in ten seconds with your eyes closed while eating a sandwich. Everything's a lot easier when you know what's coming your way—when you've played the level before.

When Henry Cejudo was preparing to fight Demetrious Johnson for the second time (he had been knocked out in the first round in their first meeting), we spent a ton of time analyzing film. We also had a professor from Arizona State University prepare some statistics that enabled us to really zero in and analyze Johnson's tendencies on a technical level. Then we brought in a bunch of training partners to simulate everything that Johnson was likely to do and ran Henry through thousands of reps so that he could anticipate and counter all of Johnson's movements. Those counters enabled Henry to create his own offense, and by the time the fight neared, Henry had essentially already fought and defeated Johnson a thousand times.

When we do these things a thousand times in training, the fighter learns to anticipate movements in that same way. So even though their first fight ended in a first-round knockout, those thousand reps gave Henry such a familiarity with his opponent he remarked that after the fight he felt like he'd already been in there with him. Much of that is a visual and psychological thing, but drilling technique in that manner that many times also created muscle memory. Henry was so reactive that he didn't even have to think about things very much because he had simulated so many of the techniques that we suspected Johnson might do (and actually did). And the result of the second fight was Henry's hand raised as the new UFC Flyweight champion of the world.

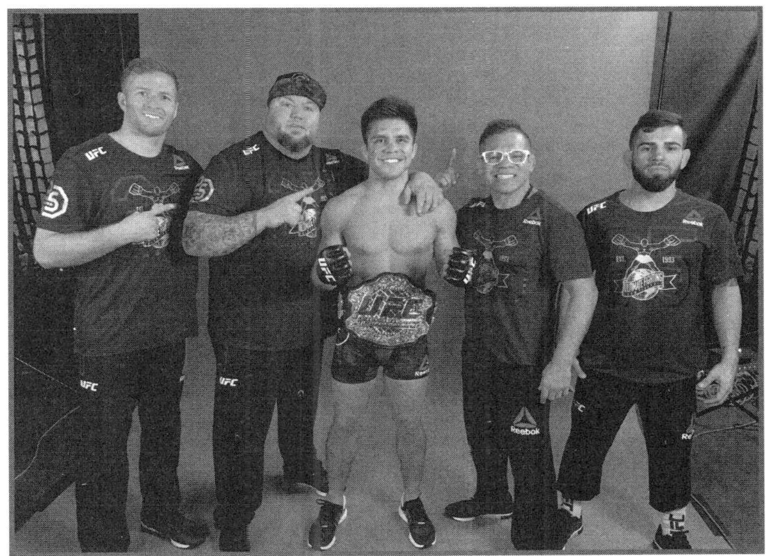

Henry was so prepared for his fight with TJ Dillashaw that the fight lasted a little over a minute before Henry won his first title defense. *Seigher Brown*

Two-time Super Bowl champion quarterback Eli Manning is someone who knows and has benefitted from the power of preparation, too. In an interview for his former head coach Tom Coughlin's 2013 book, *Earn the Right to Win*, he said, "Preparation is addictive. There is no better feeling in the world than coming up to the line of scrimmage on third down, looking at the way the defense is set up, and knowing not only exactly what they are going to do, but that you have the perfect play to counter that. Once you've experienced that feeling of calling signals totally confident that you are running the perfect play, you want to get back there again and again. You see how all the hard work you've done on the practice field, all the hours you've spent studying, and all the preparation you've done come together at that one moment and make the game look simple. The more work you do, the more the game slows down."

You may not be a UFC fighter or an NFL player, but you, too, can reap the benefits of preparation and win, to paraphrase Sun Tzu, every battle before it's fought.

WHEN YOU DON'T PREPARE, BE PREPARED TO FAIL

It takes years, if not decades, to get to a point in sports where you're able to medal—to be competitive enough to stand on the podium. Even if you're not competing professionally, the odds of winning a city marathon or local golf tournament are pretty low. The odds of winning the local swimsuit competition or bodybuilding competition with twenty competitors in your class is difficult. It almost doesn't matter how small the talent pool is. If you're competing, chances are the person next to you has been competing longer. Years of dedication go into each competition before you're even hoping to stand atop the competitive mountain in your sport. And yet, so many competitors at all levels and throughout all sports are still hitting the starting line unprepared. Most don't even know how unprepared they are, and the ones who actually do know tend to panic, as that knowledge manifests into anxiety—performance anxiety. Remember, we can only focus on the things we can control! Focusing on the past leads to guilt. Focusing on the future leads to anxiety. Focus on the now, and do what you can do—which you can only perform in the now! Yet, so many athletes go into a race without adequate miles under their belts. They race without a running coach teaching them how to periodize their training. They're overtrained and exhausted when they get to the starting line. Too many fighters are at gyms with coaches who don't know how to get their fighters the right fights and have never cut weight. If you want to win, you need to be prepared. Unfortunately, we can't just decide to "win." We have to go through all the motions just like everyone else. Even the special ones have to do things the right way, so you have to as well.

One of the easiest ways to circumvent *some* of the "learn by trial and error" method is to surround yourself with coaches and athletes who have walked your proverbial footsteps before you.

THOSE WHO CAN'T, TEACH

George Bernard Shaw wrote in "Maxims for Revolutionists," "He who can, does; He who cannot, teaches." And, although it's somewhat of a play on Aristotle's original quote "Those who know, do; those who understand, teach," there's a lot to take from it.

One of the first steps to success whether in sports or in business is to surround yourself with mentors, teachers, and coaches who can help you along your journey. If you want to open a new business, you can go online and find countless influencer accounts telling you how to market your business, how to get rich in real estate, and how to arbitrage a currency to make it rich. There are countless books and websites that say similar things. You could get lost for days and weeks diving into each, and then spend your life's savings to implement the plans in them . . . only to realize they were scams and talking points. The only one getting rich off any of the ideas is the influencer and author—by selling the courses—not by actually implementing the tactics. You fell victim to a marketing ploy, as did so many others.

What you really want is to seek out someone who's actually successful. Someone who's created a business from the ground up. Someone who's managed marketing campaigns or spent millions on Facebook and Google ad spends. And although it's probably not as glamorous as the Instagram influencers make it out to be (and certainly not as simple), there's actual substance there.

The same goes for coaches in athletics. As a youth, you probably learned first by someone's father, who happened to be the youth wrestling or football coach. Maybe he won a state championship as an athlete or at least played all four years in high school. Then, you get to high school and college, and the coaches have progressively gotten more accolades. A college player or D-I All-American. But there's experience there. The coaches and teams and staff have a proven track record of success. Those are the coaches you need to seek out. In most sports it's pretty easy to discern between those who can and the snake oil salesman, but beware!

After Henry Cejudo won the Olympic Gold medal in freestyle wrestling in 2008, he wasn't certain what his future wrestling plans were going to be. While training for the 2008 Olympics, he lived and trained at the Olympic Training Center in Colorado Springs, Colorado. He trained as the other athletes did: drilled wrestling techniques, wrestled live, ran, lifted weights. Nothing wild. Nothing novel. Just hard work. But after the 2008 Olympics, he was exhausted with wrestling, and after two books and a play were written about him, he didn't have the same focus. And here's where it gets interesting—he met someone who told him he wouldn't have to wrestle at all to prepare for the 2012 Olympics. All he had to do was run—use his patented running program—and that would prepare him to wrestle. Well, it didn't, and Henry lost at the Olympic trials and retired there on the mats.

We see snake oil salesmen all over the place—in nutrition, in MMA and boxing gyms, as strength and conditioning coaches. "I know a different way. I know an easier way. Come follow me." It's almost ubiquitous in MMA and boxing. It's literally why I decided to write this book. But it's not always snake oil we need to watch out for. Sometimes the good intentions of those who just don't know get in the way too.

"The road to hell is paved with good intentions."

Intentions aside, you need a coach who knows what he's doing. Do you want a general to take you into battle who hasn't fought on the front lines himself? Do you want business advice from someone who's only read books? No. And you want your coaches to have actual experience—whether through competition themselves or through prior success.

Choosing early coaches and gyms and teams is paramount to future development and success, as it distinguishes between what actually works and the theoretical.

As a coach to high level fighters, I see young fighters warming up before they enter the cage, and I can tell when someone from a small gym is about to get knocked out in front of everyone he knows. I can tell that his karate instructor convinced him that he could prepare the young student to fight in the cage, and in reality, he couldn't. When I go to Brazilian Jiu Jitsu competitions, I can tell who's training out of their garage with a fraud versus someone who's at a legitimate gym.

Don't take the easy route. Don't take the cheap route. The tiny dojo in the strip mall is only $99 a month because you aren't going to learn what you need from them. If you pay a real registered dietician, it's going to cost a lot more than someone's friend who's a meal prepper and will put together your diet. The strength coach at Exos is better than the guy with the big biceps at the local gym. Don't find a shortcut because the long route is too hard or expensive.

Early in my MMA journey, I'd see so many instructional DVDs titled *Beat Jiu Jitsu with Catch Wrestling* or *How to beat the Gracies with Kung Fu* or a hundred other similar titles. And those titles existed because Brazilian Jiu Jitsu is hard. The average black belt spends nearly ten years on the mats before being promoted to the rank. Don't ever "Beat X with Y." Get good at X.

If preparation is key to competition, finding the early trainers and coaches who are verified is more important than almost anything else you will ever do to prepare for competition. A good coach will guide you through your training, diet, weight cut, and more. She will be able to tell you if a new diet or strength plan seems like you should try it or run for the hills instead.

Find a doer. Find a teacher who knows.

If you do find the right person for the early stages of your career, you're going to have the right fundamentals in place.

I don't know how to train for an Ironman event. I may be able to read up on how to train. I may be able to fake a good portion of the training. I may even pull the wool over the eyes of those who have completed Ironman events before, but if you want to be competitive, I will do nothing but harm, and those who know would sniff me out fast! And you want someone who actually knows. Someone who can tell you that on mile 25 on the bike your tailbone hurts, and by mile 2 on the swim, you start shivering uncontrollably (both of those are completely made up things, by the way!). But those who know, know. And they can share the tiniest of details.

I can tell new fighters that they have never felt nerves and an adrenaline dump like they'll experience in MMA. "Oh, so you have a thousand wrestling matches under your belt? You're still going to have an adrenaline dump!" I can tell people that on my way to the cage I notice what people are wearing and what's on their shirt. I tell them that as soon as I take off my shirt at the cage I feel cold. Like shivering cold . . . regardless of how hot it is in the arena. How time stands still when the MC begins announcing your names—I always just think "shut the hell up and let's fight already!" And I know that, no matter how much "someone wants it," if they're in the middle of an adrenaline dump, it doesn't matter what we do or say, the fighter's body won't move how we want it to. You can't fake that. If you haven't been in there numerous times at a high level, you don't know those things. Knowledge is learned. Wisdom is experienced.

Go seek a wise coach from the beginning, and you're going to be much better off throughout your entire career.

And, above all, the best shortcut is hard work.

MAN IN THE MIRROR

Before you can analyze an opponent or develop a game plan, you need to fully understand your own strengths and weaknesses. As a fighter, are you a power puncher or a cardio machine? As a marathon runner, are you a fast starter or do you excel in the middle or end? As a business owner, are you a great marketer, or is operations your forte? If you don't have these basic understandings, you're setting yourself up for failure.

> *Know thyself and you will win all battles.*
>
> *—Lao Tzu (Chinese philosopher)*

First, understanding yourself means knowing what you're good at. Vince Lombardi famously quipped, "The best defense is a good offense." High-powered offenses score and score often and they take up a lot of time of possession, which leaves less time for the other team to have the ball and, therefore, score.

Now, forget about game-planning for a second and just think about showing up to the event, zero planning. How will you actually win? It seems like a simple question, but so many fighters I've trained have no idea what they are good at. Some think they have a great jab when, in reality, it's their low kick that shines. Others fancy themselves as strikers, but have five submission wins and zero knockouts. Shaq knew to stay under the rim and dunk. Steph Curry knows to shoot three pointers. And they don't confuse the two.

Lombardi understood the importance of a good offense. He understood putting the opponent on the back foot, on the defensive, would make his coaching life easier, but just stating "good offense" is too general of a concept. Macro level "good" is made up of various "micro" level components. It's the details that make the difference. I always tell my fighters that anyone on the planet can throw a jab-cross-hook combination, but the difference between someone off the street throwing their right and left hand is very different than an amateur fighter performing the same combination. And the difference between a professional performing the same combination and a Floyd Mayweather or Canelo Álvarez is light-years different too. But why? They're all doing the same macro level movement, right? Yes, but it's the details that make all the difference. Little details; big difference.

The same goes for Vince Lombardi and his offense. What made it "good"? Was it the offensive line? Was it the quarterback? And what made that O-line impenetrable? Was it their physical strength? Hand fighting? Formation? Were they great at creating holes for the running back or could they create two more seconds during the passing game for the quarterback to get the ball to the best receiver? Each detail can be broken down into a myriad of smaller, finer details. Understanding the nuances between each level of detail helps separate the mediocre from the good, and the great from the GOATs.

All sports are the same. You can break down your own offense and skills and physicality to numerous levels. Start doing so. What are you waiting for? As a fighter, I knew I wasn't the physically strongest. So, I had to be the matador, not the bull. I had to slide around people and take their back and choke them. I wasn't going to knock people out. I knew that. And I didn't waiver from what I knew I was good at. What are you good at? When the game is on the line, how are you going to win? Are you going to charge the lane and go for the dunk or get open and drop a three-pointer? When the last mile of the race is in front of you and you look to your right and there's a runner next to you, are you going to pace her and sprint the last 100 meters or are you going to fly out in front and lead? If you can't answer those self-reflective questions accurately, how do you expect to win? How can you even think of winning? Winning doesn't come from the magnitude of desire to win, it comes from the preparation to win. Fine tuning the details and techniques to perfection and focus during competition lead to winning. Remember, winning is the successful outcome to doing the details well in the moment.

If you don't know what you're good at, how can a coach train you? How can you train you? You're lost somewhere, and you need to create a map of skills and weaknesses and plot yourself on it so you can know where that elusive treasure lies.

EVEN THE DEATH STAR HAD A WEAKNESS

Most of us have seen *Star Wars*. We know the Death Star—Darth Vader's planet-sized destroyer and regulator of the galaxies. It was 99.99% indestructible. Just that one TINY opening "the size of a womp rat" that didn't have a defense system over it that could destroy the entire ship if shot at the right angle. The Death Star had a weakness in its defenses! The Terminator could be melted! If even the strongest villains on our favorite movies have weaknesses, you have one too—more likely than not, you have many weaknesses. What are they? What is your biggest weakness? If you can't answer that without asking others, you're in for a world of disappointment, and it's time to do some self-reflection—not only in athletics, but in life. If you really expect to excel, you'd better be able to answer the job interview question, "What was one of your weaknesses at your last job?" And it better not be, "Sometimes I'm just too hard of a worker" or "I'm a perfectionist."

As we spar with fighters we land a leg kick or two, and we immediately learn whether they are going to check (defend) the kicks. If they don't, we keep kicking. We do the same with jabs. The same with takedowns and submissions. We can see the weaknesses in other people so well, but sometimes we have a hard time pointing the mirror at ourselves when we train. But we need to. Just as we need to recognize patterns to learn new moves and motions as we fight, we need to recognize when we're getting hit with the same punch over and over again. Are we more tired than our training partners or our opponents in competition? Do they feel significantly stronger than us? Faster? Do we keep getting caught in the same submission?

We need to know which bricks are loose in our great walls because we need to know where improvements should be made. But we also need to know our weaknesses, so we know where our opponents are going to attack. If we have a weakness, and then work on raising that skill, now we have a "perceived weakness" that an opponent may try to exploit, which may bring on our own counterattack if we're prepared.

The strongest offense is such a waste of talent if there's a weakness so great, it can take the whole platoon down. We see fighters all the time with the most gorgeous boxing and power punching in the sport only to see them end up taken down and submitted and offer little to zero on the mat. Losses pile up, and we say, "What if?"

TIME TO STUDY

I'm not sure I see any sports utilizing film study as much as American football. My thirteen-year-old son's first-year tackle team has multiple film sessions a week—and they're mandatory if any of the kids want playing time. In the NFL tape-study is ubiquitous. You HAVE to watch film. There are only so many hours a day that you can play ball and watch different defenses and schemes and fakes and motions in person, on the field. The NFL is so advanced and nuanced. Without film, it'd take a player ten lifetimes to understand what was in front of him. But through tape study, as a receiver, you can see how the cornerback stutters his left foot when he's planning press coverage and how he clenches his fists when he's blitzing. You can see how the motion man sets off a jet sweep or five other plays from the same motion. You have to see the patterns again and again. You must understand how your opponent plays the game—on both offense and defense. If you go in blind and just start picking plays, it's a coin toss whether you come out the victor or not, but in reality, the odds are probably significantly stacked against you. It's like playing against someone with a crystal ball in front of them reading the future, while you're playing with a blindfold over your eyes.

The MMA community has traditionally not watched a ton of film. However, coaches and fighters are beginning to watch more film more regularly. Honestly, I think I probably watch too much film—as I study approximately 5–10 hours of film a week. And I already told you about how we brought in Kevin Grimm, a tenured Arizona State University professor, to run stats on Demetrious Johnson when Henry Cejudo rematched him for the UFC Flyweight belt. Kevin holds the rank of full professor at ASU, and has his PhD in psychology and teaches classes in Statistics, Longitudinal Growth Modeling, Structural Equation Modeling, and more—he might have been a bit overskilled for our needs!

We needed to know how easy it was for people to back Demetrious up into the fence. How many times Demetrious threw a knee off the break when he shot for a takedown and his opponent defended (31%), and how often he threw a knee when his opponents shot a takedown, but he defended (42%). How often did Demetrious begin his punching combinations with a straight right hand (79%)? Knowing this information was paramount in beating Demetrious. We could have watched tape on our own, but as humans, we have confirmation bias—we see what we want to see. We want to see what we're looking for. We have biases. Hiring an outside statistician to run the numbers took away what we "thought" DJ did in his fights and told us exactly what he "did" in his fights.

I don't expect most of you reading this to go hire a statistician for every competition. We paid over $9,000 per breakdown, and that's just not feasible for most people. But you can watch film and note trends. But don't watch and stare and expect to remember everything—just like in social studies class in middle school, take notes! Write down what you see in film if you notice it more than once. Then create hash marks for each time you see it again. Then go back and see what trends (both offensively and defensively) are more prevalent. Make sure to do this for both strengths and weaknesses.

Try to look at macro- and micromovements. An example of a macromovement is watching an opponent throw a jab and then level change into a double leg takedown. The micro-level movement would be whether he steps through the double leg with his lead leg or if he steps through with his rear leg. Does he lift opponents off the ground or drop to a knee and turn the corner? In basketball, you'd want to recognize an offensive pattern, such as Phil Jackson's famous triangle offense, but you may need to recognize a specific movement of how a player pivots off a left foot when he shoots vs his right foot when he tends to pass the ball. Both are equally important in their own way.

FITTING THE SQUARE PEG IN THE SQUARE HOLE

Game planning is more puzzle work than science. You wouldn't try to shove a square peg in a round hole. We give that game to our infants, and they get it right after a few tries, so why are you trying to smash down an opponent's weakness with a "non-strength" of your own? Each puzzle piece has its correct place, and you can't try to force it in where it doesn't fit.

Don't look so closely and narrowly at something that you see the trees, but not the forest.

I use football analogies a lot—even with my fighters (even those fighters who don't know the NFL). Giving context to a move in a different sport allows for fighters to get out of their own head and look at things from a different point of view. Football seems the easiest for everyone to understand, as most know the sport well enough to comprehend, but there are such clearly defined roles in football that it's easy to break down. And each play is only a few seconds, and then there's a reset button for it to start again and again.

Now that we have our film study, we know exactly what our opponent does well and poorly. We know how often he does it. And we know what we're good at and poor at. Both sides are analyzed. Let the planning begin!

Back to the square peg.

Too often, I see fighters and coaches trying to exploit weaknesses at all costs. But it's not always that easy. You need to match strengths for weaknesses, and if that doesn't work out, strength for strength. But don't try to exploit an opponent with a weakness of your own team or fighter, or even a "non-strength" (being okay at something, but maybe not good), unless there is absolutely no other option.

Now, let's play a game: You're calling the offense for the Tampa Bay Buccaneers, and you're facing the weak defensive line of the Carolina Panthers. Well, you may want to smash the run game down their throat, but what if your star running back is injured and your backup has been horrible the last few games? That doesn't make any sense. But you have Mike Evans, a future Hall of Fame wide receiver, and they have a rookie cornerback and a weak safety—throw that ball to Mike every single play!

But what if the scenario is the same, but instead of a rookie cornerback, you have an all pro? And there's even a good safety in the secondary too? I say throw that ball to Mike Evans and see if he can come down with it. Go strength for strength as much as possible. If it's not working as much as you hoped, get another receiver in the area to pull coverage off Mike Evans and throw that ball up again. I'd much rather play to my strengths, even if they are my opponent's strengths, than try to exploit a weakness with a weakness. But the key is finding the right peg for the hole. The easiest way I've found to do this is to go old-school and draw on a wipe board each fighter's (3–4) strengths and weaknesses, and then line up what seems like it will cancel out or be an advantage/disadvantage.

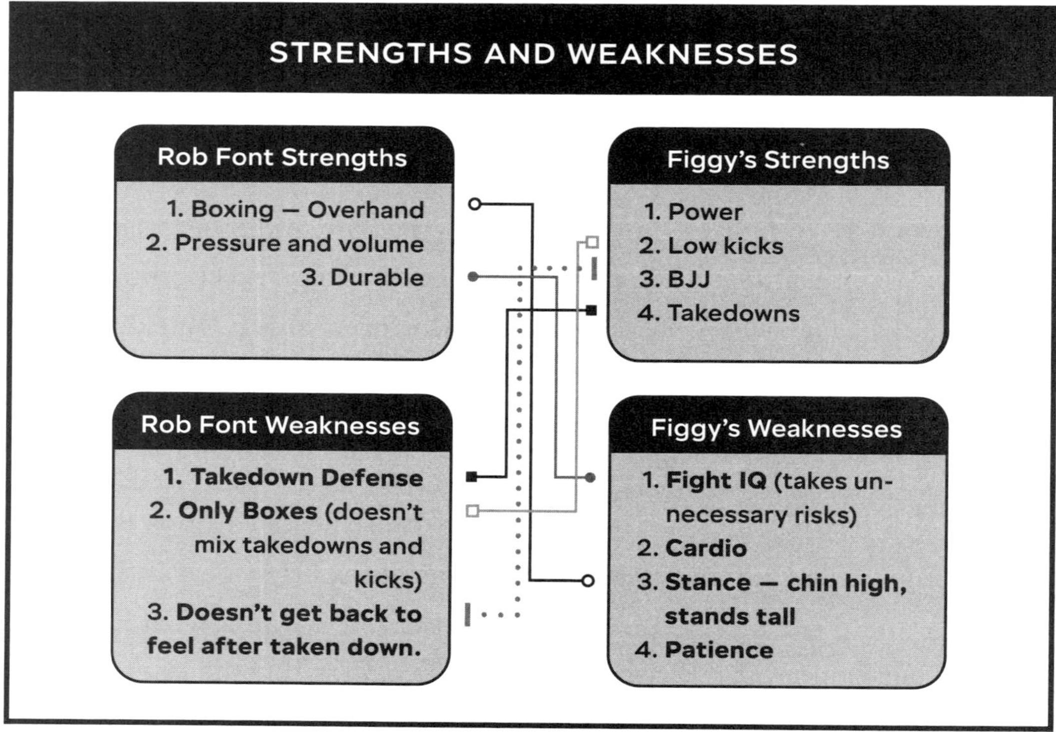

On the previous page is an actual list of how we broke down Deiveson Figueiredo's strengths and weaknesses when he moved up a weight class to fight Rob Font at a UFC Fight Night in Austin, Texas, on Dec. 2, 2023.

A lot of Figgy's strengths matched up with Rob's weaknesses, so that was an easy offensive game plan to work toward. Figgy has good leg kicks, good takedowns, and good grappling. We knew with Rob's stance we could kick his leg. We knew we could get the takedown, and we knew that once on the ground, Figgy could control and find some strikes and create some damage.

Where we were concerned was with Figgy's tendency to lose focus and take unnecessary risks and Font's durability. We worried if Figgy couldn't get Font out early, he'd start taking unnecessary risks that might put him in bad positions. We also worried that with Figgy's tendency to hold his chin high, Font would land his own overhand right and connect with/hurt Figgy.

The owner of our gym runs these meetings and has us rank each strength and weakness 1–10. One being bad; ten being the best. With the weaknesses, we work on trying to bring from, say, a two or a three out of ten to a six/seven/eight out of ten. We must have an offense AND a defense, just like in the NFL.

Fortunately, our game plan worked for Figgy with this fight, and he won a unanimous decision and dominated Rob Font—allowing him to climb the ranks of his new division.

BRAINS VS BRAWN

You're the perfect student. You asked all the right questions. You had perfect attendance. You studied. You practiced. You now have the best mind in the game . . . but that big, strong guy with the unlimited cardio just smashed you!

This happens more than you think in fighting; the better fighter doesn't always win. It happens in other sports too. Just look at the third period or fourth quarter of any team sport—hockey, football, basketball, soccer—as fatigue sets in, big plays happen. Teams come back from behind to snatch defeat out of the grips of opponents and small leads turn to massive deficits.

One of the million sayings I repeat to my fighters is "It doesn't matter who's better, it matters who comes off the stool fresher for round two."

Conditioning is key, and there's a strange balancing act between technical abilities and conditioning. The technical disparity between two fighters significantly changes the role of strength and conditioning. If fighter A is so much better than fighter B, B probably won't make it into the second round. Fighter A is winning by submission or knockout in round one. But if fighter A is, say, 80% better than fighter B, then A's conditioning probably just has to be good enough to get through round two and so on. But if fighter A is barely more technical than fighter B, say it's a 55%–45% split, then fighter A better be well-conditioned because, depending on fighter B's conditioning level, the tides could change. Now, let's flip it. Fighter A is not the technically superior fighter, well, he just needs to be good enough to get into round two, and if his conditioning is significantly superior, he can take over the fight and win rounds two and three. The closer the skill level, or if you're operating at a technical deficiency, the greater the role cardio, and to a lesser degree, strength and power, will have on the outcome of the fight (or competition).

It's very common to see a fighter win round one by a huge margin, gas out, and lose round two and three or get finished because her cardio failed. And, we need to note, sometimes cardio isn't cardio at all, but is significantly affected by adrenaline—due to inexperience, or maybe a fighter almost finished his opponent and went for the kill, only for his opponent to stave off the attack. Adrenaline dumps have probably been the cause of more "cardio collapses" than all the cardio training in the world could equate to, in MMA, at least.

I'll discuss strength and conditioning in full in part two of this book, but it is equally as important as technique and honestly, for some fighters, it's way more important than technique. There's no perfect recipe for a fighter or linebacker or power forward. There's a balancing act of speed, strength, power, technique, flexibility, sight, predictive abilities, intelligence, and a hundred other traits that make up a good athlete. All we can do is train each to the best of our abilities.

SCHEDULING IS A MUST

There is, however, one more thing to mention during the preparation phase for a fighter or any athlete: scheduling. You must, and I cannot express *must* enough, create a weekly schedule. Below, you'll see two actual training schedules of fighters we've run camps for.

On the next page, you see Zhang Weili's schedule when she rematched Rose Namajunas for the women's Flyweight title. Note that the intensity of each workout varies, with the lighter days preceding sparring days, which should be the most difficult workout at the highest intensity each week.

On page 103, you'll see Amir Albazi's schedule for a fight that actually got canceled due to an emergency neck surgery needed by Amir. The schedule below is different than the one above—each needs to be personalized for each athlete, but the importance cannot be overstated. Scheduling is important to ensure all of the bases are being covered. Technical training, sparring, strength, and conditioning. Not only does each coach and athlete know when to show up, and with whom he will be working, but there are only so many hours in a day and the body needs recovery and regulation. Without a carefully planned training schedule, overtraining is almost guaranteed—much of which can be blamed on the anxiety of not working hard enough and the need to ensure no stone has been left unturned. Without planning, it's difficult to discern whether enough work is being put in. With a training schedule, everything can be monitored and measured—and adjusted if needed!

ZHANG WEILI'S SCHEDULE						
	MONDAY	TUESDAY	WEDNESDAY	THURSDAY	FRIDAY	SATURDAY
9:00	Wrestling/BJJ 6-7/10	Mitts/Striking 5-6/10		Wrestling/BJJ 6-7/10	Mitts/Striking 5-6/10	
9:30						
10:00						
10:30						
11:00						
11:30						
12:00			Sparring 9-10/10			Sparring 9-10/10
12:30						
1:00						
1:30						
2:00		POD			POD	Cryo/Recovery
2:30						
3:00						
3:30						
4:00						
4:30						
5:00	S&C 7-8/10	Soft tissue work/Recovery	Mitts/striking 7-8/10	S&C 7-8/10	Soft tissue work/Recovery	
5:30						
6:00						
6:30						

Note: All workouts are coordinated for optimal performance on sparring day. Maximizing performance of sparring is the main weekly goal, as that is the closest to a fight we will experience. The days before sparring are "lighter" to help with this peak performance.

Also, note workouts are coded by intensity. 1 being the lowest, and 10 being the most intense.

AMIR'S TRAINING SCHEDULE

	MONDAY	TUESDAY	WEDNESDAY	THURSDAY	FRIDAY	SATURDAY	SUNDAY
9:00	Santino						
10:00	10am / shootboxing	Eddie	Sparring / 10am	Eddie / Santino	Drilling / Review		
11:00					Everyone	Sparring at 11	
12:00							
1:00							
2:00							
3:00							
4:00							
5:00	Boxing Mitts						
6:00	45-1hr Aerobic	45-1hr Aerobic	45-1hr Aerobic	45-1hr Aerobic	45-1hr Aerobic		
7:00	S and C / Dan	S and C / Dan	S and C / Dan	S and C / Dan	S and C / Dan		
Intensity							
Volume							

Note that the level of intensity could be arbitrary, depending on your sport and training regimen, but our team usually uses a heart rate monitor, which allows us to monitor exactly how hard our athlete's body is working and for how long. Heart rate monitors help us keep track of workload, intensity, duration, and rest duration. They also help to diagnose overtraining symptoms as well, but we'll get into heart rate monitors later.

5

HOW TO HANDLE INJURIES AND SETBACKS

The saying "it's not how hard you fall, it's how high you bounce" has been repeated so often that it's become a cliché, but there's a kernel of truth in every cliché. With the razor-thin margin for error professional mixed martial artists face, even the very best are likely to get humbled. Setbacks in MMA don't always occur in the ring, nor as losses. Sometimes they're about injury sustained during training, an unforeseen illness, difficulty making weight, or something that transpires in a fighter's personal life.

I arrived in Boston the day before the fight—a Friday. Our team's striking coach, Eddie Cha, and our other fighter, Hunter Azure, flew out earlier in the week with Jonathan Pearce, who was making his UFC debut against the wildly popular Bostonian, Joe Lauzon. The fight was up a weight class at lightweight, but JP loved the matchup, as Lauzon was getting older and was known predominantly as a grappler. I wanted one of the fights the promotion offered us at Featherweight, but once the fight was booked at 155 lb. against Lauzon, there's no turning back and there's no wavering—fighting takes 100 percent focus and confidence from everyone in camp.

The next day, we went down for the pre-fight shakeout. We always get a quick workout on the morning of a fight—nothing long. Just enough to break a sweat, get the lungs breathing heavy, and spiking the heart rate. The reasons for the shakeout are many, and I'll go over them further in the strength and conditioning section a bit later.

"How are you feeling, JP?" I asked as we arrived in the workout room.

"Hey, who should I call out after I win tonight? I was thinking Diego Sanchez or even Charles Rosa back down at 145," he said with his thick Tennessee drawl, half ignoring my question, as he already had something on his mind.

"Let's focus on tonight first, JP," Eddie said.

We left the workout room after about thirty minutes of shadowboxing, mitt work, and wrestling. The evening's warm-up would be very similar, if not replicate completely what we just did.

In the evening, at the fight arena, during the same workout, JP turned and said, "I'm not even nervous for this fight. No nerves at all." My heart sank into my stomach.

The fight was only 93 seconds long. JP didn't only lose, he got TKO'd. Maybe worse, though, he tore numerous ligaments in his shoulder and was out of training and fighting for nearly nine months. Not exactly how he expected, or hoped, his UFC debut would play out.

There's a lot to unpack here with the JP situation.

First, it shows how you can never overlook an opponent. JP was more concerned with his in-cage callout on the microphone after the fight than he was the actual fight. He was "excited just to be there," which is never a good outlook on competition. You don't want to make it to the UFC, you want to win in the

UFC. You don't want to be invited to a football tryout; you want to make the team. You want to WIN the race, not run in the race.

Second, we want nerves. They're earned. Nerves mean you care about things. We aren't nervous for what we don't care about. More on both of those points later.

Last, was JP's shoulder injury a fluke, or could he have avoided it? If he could have avoided it, how? Whether he could have avoided the injury or not, JP could have definitely taken a different approach to training that might have mitigated the injury. But there was a silver lining. After the loss, JP started focusing on lifting weights and becoming more athletic. He always had good cardio, but it seemed like he wasn't strong or tough enough to push his opponents to a point where he could use his superior conditioning as an advantage. By dedicating himself to lifting weights, he was able to transform himself physically. After being humbled on national television, Jonathan also realized that he needed to improve on a technical level if he was going to be able to compete against the veteran fighters in the UFC. That meant returning to his fighting roots, which is wrestling. He really honed those skills and became a much better fighter in the process. It was a remarkable transformation, but it might not have happened had he not lost his debut against Lauzon. The likelihood is that he'd be 2–2 or maybe 3–3 in the UFC and be out, cut already. But instead, he went on a five-fight winning streak and found himself ranked in the top 15, and I believe his humiliating loss to Lauzon was the catalyst that helped transform him into the fighter he is today.

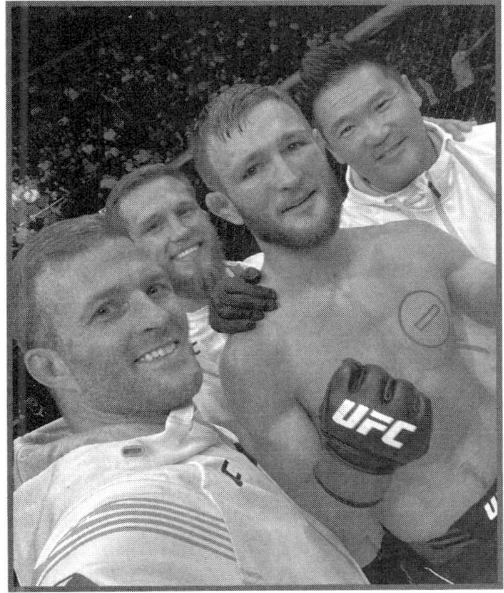

JP was set back over a year, but there's always a silver lining in losses and injuries. *Seigher Brown*

SO MANY INJURIES, SO LITTLE TIME

One of the most common setbacks an athlete will face comes in the form of injuries. They happen in the cage or on the field. They happen in training. They happen playing catch with a child or basketball with friends on the court. Hell, some people have hurt themselves on the way to the cage or gotten into car accidents on fight week! Some are minor and require a short time-out, while others can keep you out of the cage for a year or longer, or worse, end a career.

FIRST STEP: PREVENTION

There are numerous steps athletes can take to prevent injuries:

Proprioception training

- **Enhancement of athletic performance**
  - Proprioception is the "rub your stomach and pat your head at the same time" type of training that athletes need in loads to perform well. It's understanding the "feel" of a movement. Proprioceptors are little sensors in the body's ligaments, muscles, and tendons. Proprioceptive training programs focusing on balance and coordination reduced the risk of certain injuries by **50%,** according to a systematic review in the *Journal of Athletic Training.*

- **Reduction of injury risk**
  - In lower limb sports injuries (ACL/meniscus tears), proprioception exercises reduced injury occurrence by **40%** in controlled trials.

Proprioception training might take the form of one-leg squats or lunges or balancing on an unstable platform. Ropes and cables are a great way to add instability to surfaces to force athletes to balance differently—while performing weight training or athletic training. Gymnasts—in virtually every facet of sports—tend to have great proprioception. One way to improve proprioception is by doing things you're not great at—try walking on your hands, or performing a back handspring. Try things that are physically difficult for you to perform—these types of movements increase proprioception and are great ways to increase myelin in the brain, which is talked about at length in *The Talent Code*. But just be aware, once you become good at those same movements, they don't have the same effect on the mind-body connection and will need to be replaced with other activities you're not good at.

Strength training

- **Preventative effects**
  - Strength training reduced acute injuries by **33%** and overuse injuries by **50%** in a meta-analysis in the *British Journal of Sports Medicine*.

- **Injury-risk relationship**
  - Athletes who completed more than **80%** of their planned strength training sessions had an overall reduction in injuries by **20–30%** compared to those who skipped sessions.

Show me an athlete who doesn't lift, and I'll hold your ear hostage for an hour and rant on all of the reasons why she won't be a successful professional. In MMA, of course, there's the obvious reasons: while battling people in hand-to-hand competition the stronger woman has a strength advantage, generally a muscular endurance advantage, and a neuromuscular advantage to stimulus, but maybe the biggest is that she actually makes it to the fight because she's more durable and didn't get injured during training camp!

There's a story of Yoel Romero, an Olympic silver medalist in freestyle wrestling who went on to fight for a UFC title at middleweight. He is a colossus. Google him and be mystified by the trap muscles that triangulate from his shoulders to his ears. A product of the Cuban wrestling system, in 2011 he was training and felt a "crack" in his neck. He went to the doctor and found that one of his vertebrae was severely broken. The lore is that his muscles and tendons were so thick due to his years of wrestling that they were the only thing keeping him from being permanently paralyzed—being so strong, they kept his neck from breaking completely. Now, I'm not sure about all of that, but we do know that Yoel's neck and traps are bigger than any other fighter I've ever seen (maybe Brock Lesnar might have him beat), and he credits them for being the reason he is still able to walk.

You may not need neck-saving traps, but do you want to be the guy on the football field who deadlifts 500 lb. or the guy who just uses "body weight" exercises and is really technical and flexible? Exactly.

Now, there is an asterisk here!

Although lifting is great at preventing injuries, you want to make sure it isn't the CAUSE of your injuries. Proper form and proper load are imperative for not only strength gains, but also injury prevention too.

Some of my fighters used to train with a guy we'll call "Chad" (because that's his name). He came from a football background and was completely old-school. His motto was "lift these heavy things as many times as you can and then lift those heavy things as many times as you can." Training load be damned. Technique be damned. "Those things are trivial and we're here lifting now!" was his type of attitude. And, honestly, as much as he disliked me (I always suggested other S&C [strength and conditioning] coaches due to the loads he programmed), his guys were always better conditioned than the S&C coaches who had the "safety first" attitude. But the athletes who worked with him were always dead. They were so sore they could barely get through skills training. They were injured all the time. Hell, his son had some major rhabdomyolysis symptoms (a condition where there are too many toxins in the bloodstream—generally caused by overtraining in athletes) numerous times due to the high training volumes. So, more isn't always better.

Sleep

- **Role in recovery and injury prevention**
  - I spoke about sleep earlier. Its importance cannot be overstated. Go to chapter 2 if you need a refresher, but proper sleep is one of the best ways you can reduce injuries.

Stretching

- **Effectiveness in injury prevention**
  - The *British Journal of Sports Medicine* found that stretching alone reduced injury risk by only **4%**, which is considered statistically insignificant.
  - Specific to muscle injuries, stretching reduced the incidence of strains by **30%** when combined with warm-ups.

So, this is a super controversial topic. *To stretch or not to stretch?* There are too many studies to list that compare stretching versus strength training for injury prevention and, yet, more studies that compare static stretching versus dynamic stretching (go to the strength chapters for details on the differences). The consensus is that strength training reduces injuries better than stretching, and dynamic stretching reduces injuries more than static stretching. Now, my issue with these is they are mutually exclusive studies and studies that focus on stretching as a warm-up to workouts. I'm not going to go into detail about these studies and statistics and the benefits of each—go to Google Scholar and have a field day—as I'm not here to prove or disprove the efficacy of stretching. What I do want to say, though, is:

1. Why not perform all three? Strength train to get strong. Dynamic stretching to warm up. Static stretching to become more flexible. I've never seen flexibility hinder an athlete; I've only seen benefits from athletes who are more flexible—in their technical abilities and in injury prevention. A more flexible athlete will move more freely than a stiffer athlete, especially when encountering unforeseen circumstances (slip on snow/wet field while running, being on a single leg and being tripped). Henry Cejudo probably wouldn't be an Olympic gold medalist if he wasn't flexible enough to withstand some insane takedown attempts, where the only thing that saved him was his flexibility. Being more flexible is only going to help you.

2. Why does all static stretching have to be in relation to a warm-up for a workout? I'm not sure if people understand this, but static stretching can be performed separate from a workout. There's nothing preventing athletes from . . . just stretching! Not as a warm-up. Not as a cooldown. Just stretching for the sake of stretching—late at night or early in the morning. In front of the TV or out in a park. Just stretch. Your body will thank you for being nimbler as a human and all of your athletic movements will be freer.

Managing workload/progressive overload

- **Importance of gradual progression**
    - Research in the *Journal of Sports Sciences* highlighted that increasing weekly training volume by more than **15%** raised the risk of overuse injuries by **28%**.

- Adhering to a gradual increase (e.g., the "10% rule") reduced injuries by **25–30%** in endurance sports.

This is the "end all, be all" of injury prevention. Athletes, calm the hell down and manage your damn workload! I usually see two versions of mismanaged workloads. The first is going from the couch to full-on training mode without a "ramp up" period. The second is the "all gas, no breaks year-round" type. The habitual overtrained—always working. Always grinding. Go. Go. Go. In both instances, it's too much too fast and the body can't handle the load—so something breaks. Maybe it's a bone or ligament. Maybe it's an immune system breakdown in the form of a sickness or staph infection. I'll speak more about "progressive overload" when we get to the strength and conditioning section. But the short is: Follow the "10% rule" (increase volume/intensity by 10% each week) or even better, the "5% rule." The issue with 10% is that athletes tend to increase weight training by 10% and then running by 10% and their sport-specific training by at least 10% (usually they just hit the gas here). And this doesn't mean add 5–10% of weight for each exercise—that's probably very unrealistic. We're talking training volume here.

Additional strategies to reduce injuries

- **Off-season management**
  - One thing I've noticed with athletes is many don't manage their off-season effectively. They go from gas to brakes to gas.
  - So often, I see fighters end a camp (the same concept applies for those who fight, run a race, play professional football, or any cyclical sport) and gain massive amounts of weight. They've spent months starving themselves eating chicken and broccoli, and then they blow

up eating ice cream and fast food for weeks on end. They don't train—either due to injury or mental fatigue or travel or [insert every excuse in the book here]. Weeks or months go by and then they get the call for another fight. They come to the gym and floor the gas pedal of intensity, and then find themselves injured—popped rib, tweaked ankle, torn ligament. Minor to major. Able to push through and fight to having to pull out and sit on the bench for months.

- When athletes maintain some semblance of athletic training and adequate nutrition programs, starting camp is so much easier—mentally, and in the form of avoiding injuries. We say, "Stay ready, so you don't have to get ready."

- **Proper nutrition and hydration**
    - Maintaining adequate hydration reduced cramping and related injuries by **20–25%**, as found in endurance sports trials.
    - Hydration is going to help with your physical performance. We know this. But it's going to help with your cognitive performance (which will translate to physical performance) as well.
    - And last but not least, nutrition. We have a whole section on this—it's why I wanted to write this whole book, so see part three for much deeper insight. But, to summarize, eating like an adult is paramount to ensuring your body is performing optimally. Eat balanced meals for 85% of your diet and do whatever you want with the other 15% (outside of strict diet training camps/needs). If you eat fast food for breakfast and lunch daily, you're getting empty calories—macronutrients (fats, carbs, proteins), but without a lot of the micronutrients (vitamins, minerals, antioxidants). Eating well is going to keep your body fat lower (huge for injury prevention), and it's going

to ensure you have the energy to perform well and the energy for your body to recover from workouts.

Common misconceptions

- **Stretching prevents all injuries**
  - I mentioned this above, but I did want to add it here, as there are some misconceptions about stretching. First, static stretching hasn't shown efficacy in reducing injuries while performed BEFORE A WORKOUT (AS A MEANS TO WARM UP). General stretching does not significantly reduce injury risk beyond the **4%,** and static stretching prior to dynamic/ballistic movements (sprinting, power cleans) has even shown a slight increase in injury risk.
  - Use static stretching as a means to become more flexible, not as a means to reduce injury.

- **Protective equipment eliminates risk**
  - Athletes wearing protective gear, such as helmets or pads, often engage in riskier behaviors, reducing the net protective effect by up to **30%.**
  - I always tell my fighters that headgear doesn't prevent brain injuries or CTE (chronic traumatic encephalopathy)—avoid getting punched in the head if that's your worry. The Olympic Boxing committee recently removed the requirement for male boxers to wear headgear during competition, as there's evidence that there's no reduction in brain injuries while wearing it. That said, headgear will help prevent eye pokes, head butts, and other weird accidents.

- Wearing the proper athletic equipment can absolutely help reduce the risk of some injuries. The issue lies with people thinking they're wearing bulletproof armor and feeling indestructible—which is where many injuries arise from. Just because you have a football helmet on doesn't mean you should be leading with your head on tackles—we recently saw the YouTube star Deestroying make his way to the UFL (a minor-league football organization) and deliver a wild tackle off of a kickoff, where he led with his head, right into a player running at full speed toward him. Deestroying left the game and it was later revealed that he had fractured a vertebra in his spine. Just because you put on a bulletproof vest, doesn't mean you should be asking people to shoot you in the chest!

Now, what none of you want to hear: Sometimes shit happens. That's right. Sometimes injuries just occur. And many times it's not the crazy stuff that does it—I always joke that me and a training partner can agree to go as hard as we can—"To the death!" and we'll come out just fine. It's when we agree to go light or "just move" when one of us gets hurt. Someone throws faster or harder than the other expects, and an injury comes out of nowhere. One of the worst injuries I ever had was when my firstborn son was about six months old, and I picked him up from his car seat and opened my trunk. I reached in nonchalantly and grabbed his stroller with my free hand, and it felt like a needle stuck my spinal cord. I could barely move for weeks. Not running or lifting or punching or kicking. Just normal dad stuff. Most recently, my wife and I feared that the same child (fourteen now) would get hurt during his first season of tackle football. He was fine, but my younger son fell during the first play of his flag-football season—which was supposed to be the "safe sport"—and reached his hand out to catch his balance. His thumb hit the ground and he tore his

UCL and fractured his thumb with the most benign-looking slip ever seen to man—it usually doesn't make sense.

Sometimes we take all the precautions in the world, but still find ourselves on the IR list (Injured Reserve list). Then it becomes about rehab and staying mentally focused. Other times we get injured and just have to push through it—because that's all we can do.

NANA KOROBI, YA OKI

Injuries are a part of sports, just as setbacks are a part of life. Nothing is linear. We've heard the saying "two steps forward, one step back." Heck, just look at the five-year line of a very good stock. Look at some of the more known ones (Tesla, Apple, Facebook, Costco—all solid at the time of writing this), and you'll see dips and valleys and peaks all over the place! But they all trend up and to the right—but not even one travels in a straight line.

There's a Japanese proverb (above) that roughly translates to "Get knocked down seven times, stand up eight." It never really made much sense to me on a literal level because the math doesn't really add up as I'm not sure the initial standing process would count, but I digress. . . . We get what it means. Don't quit when things get tough. Be resilient. Make a great comeback. Remember, everybody loves a great comeback.

Although I did talk about some ways to prevent injuries during training, on an athletic level, I'm not going to do the same for recovering from them—that's a doctor and physical therapist's job. I want to discuss the psychological side of rebounding from injuries and setbacks, as that's where I have experience—unfortunately, too much—both personally and with my fighters!

I could start with my own experience—I was a promising up and coming fighter with a record of 11–2 when I was accepted as a participant in *The Ultimate Fighter* TV show, which aired on Spike TV, pitting sixteen fighters in a house, with the winner receiving a UFC contract. A few days before filming began, the UFC president, Dana White, called me and informed me of a brain aneurysm behind my left eye, in my carotid artery. Doctors told me I'd never fight again. I underwent brain surgery, and then after two years away from the sport, I made my MMA return and eventually won enough to be accepted into the ninth season of *The Ultimate Fighter*—don't call it a comeback! But I won't go into that story here. I wrote an entirely different book chronicling that in my memoir, *There Are No Hospitals in Russia*. But it gives you a bit of insight that I'm fully aware of what it's like to be "there" one moment and then have it all disappear in an instant and to persevere through all the emotions and negativity that come with a life-changing diagnosis.

Athletic setbacks are similar to a death of a loved one. Not in terms of the severity of the situation, but how people handle the emotions that come with the setback. Most of us have heard of the stages of grief—different emotional stages people who experience loss go through: denial, anger, bargaining, depression, and acceptance. Most people experience each of those stages—not necessarily in that order and not necessarily for equal time—after a death in the family . . . but also while sidelined with injuries.

STICKS AND STONES . . .

The average bone break takes six weeks to heal. Even a broken femur, all the way through—just six weeks (barring surgeries and metal). The average ACL surgery—considered one of the worst injuries an athlete can endure, due to the recovery time—will average six months to a year. I actually have a fighter, Sheymon Moraes, who tore his ACL before a fight and returned from surgery almost six months to the day to his next fight, which took place in the Professional Fighters League cage. He won, but he probably should not have fought that soon. The body's ability to heal itself is absolutely remarkable—

next time you bite your tongue, just take note how it's almost healed by the next morning. The efficiency of the body to repair its bones and tissues and organs sometimes makes me think I'm Wolverine from the X-Men—a mutant who could heal himself from virtually any injury in lightning-fast time. But for as fast as our bodies can heal themselves, there's one organ we can't help with much: the brain. The brain is a finicky thing. We cannot repair the actual mass of the brain—the cells and synapses and matter. Our brains don't heal like the rest of our body's cells. But maybe worse, our psychology tends to have a much slower path to recovery than our bones and ligaments and tendons, and there's no amount of surgeries that can just "make our fears better."

Post-traumatic stress disorder (PTSD) isn't just for war veterans. It's for anyone who's undergone a traumatic event—and many sports injuries can create the same type of cortisone spike that burns the memories of the injury into our minds just like those in war.

On November 18, 2018, Alex Smith, quarterback for the Washington Redskins at the time, looked down to "see [his] leg bending where it shouldn't, and the realization that [his] leg was severely broken," sunk in. It was a compound fracture of his tibia and fibula, and his leg bent a way it never should.

What should have been the start of a recovery back to the NFL for Smith set off a series of surgeries and infections that left him fighting for his life, and to save his leg. The break was so bad that, initially, doctors didn't even know if they'd be able to save his leg—they were much more concerned about his ability to walk again than they were about his NFL career.

Over the course of almost a year, Smith underwent seventeen different surgeries to remove necrotizing infections and regraft bone as they worked to maintain his leg and keep it intact. His orthopedic surgeon, Dr. Robin West, said, "We were in life-saving mode now and leg-saving mode, but it's in that order." Even after the infection was under control, doctors thought Smith might still need to amputate his leg.

Postsurgeries and recovery left him needing to learn to walk, and he wondered if he'd ever play with his kids again—playing on the gridiron wasn't even being considered . . . until it was.

Somehow, someway, Alex Smith began to not only walk, but run, and running led to throwing and practicing again. "I'm saying out loud that I want to go see if I can play football again. And I was scared to death when I said it, but I wasn't scared to try." During the 2020 NFL season, Alex Smith returned to the NFL and defied every odd to have ever been placed on a sport.

There's always a mental component involved when returning to anything after injury; my children don't want to play with a toy after they bump their elbow on its side—it's a natural fear response to injury. Our physiology and psychology, built up by millennia of evolution as we try to stay alive, blocks us from engaging in risky behaviors, especially when those risky behaviors have already rendered terrifying results. But overcoming fear is the definition of courage, and you can't be courageous if you don't have fear before it. Courage without fear is just ignorance.

SOMETIMES WE DON'T HAVE TIME TO RUMINATE. ACTION IS IMMINENT

I talked about JP above—a long-term injury. Surgery after the fight. But what happens when an injury occurs during the fight? We've seen so many shoulders dislocate mid-fight—Korean Zombie's against José Aldo. TJ Dillashaw's against Aljermain Sterling. ACL ligaments torn mid-fight or on the gridiron are almost so common we expect it. But sometimes something spectacular happens.

After UFC bantamweight champion TJ Dillashaw came down to challenge Henry Cejudo for Henry's Flyweight belt (Henry won via knockout/TKO in the first round), Dillashaw tested positive for the banned substance EPO—a performance enhancing drug that helps the body develop more oxygen-transferring blood cells. He was suspended and his bantamweight title was relinquished. Henry chose to move up a weight class and fight the tough Marlon Moraes for the vacant title.

Henry took a beating during the first round of their fight, mostly on his legs via kicks, but overall, it was rough. He adjusted in the second and pressed forward and took control with his boxing. The tides were turning. But when he came back to the stool after round two, he told me, "I hurt my right shoulder. Bad. I can't use it anymore."

"Can you use your left?" I asked.

"Yeah," he responded.

"You need to crowd him and smother him with pressure," I said. "Clinch him and wrestle him."

And he did. Henry clinched him and landed knee after knee to Marlon's head. Eventually Henry dropped him and swarmed, getting the TKO.

But there was never quit in Henry. I've been in too many corners to know when someone wants out of a fight—when they are looking for an excuse. So often winners don't win fights, instead the losers quit—whether by actually quitting or just quitting in the moments, which leads to the overall loss. But champions don't have that quit switch. Henry didn't. We were playing chess, not checkers—his queen was taken, so he had to use his rook to do the job. It's the people who refuse to acknowledge the option of ever quitting—even when times get difficult, whether caused by injury or fluke or a hurricane or act of God—who get their names written. Who get their names remembered.

6

NERVES ARE EARNED

MMA is a tough sport for tough competitors, but everybody who competes in the sport—from beginners to world champions—gets nervous before a fight. Instead of telling my fighters not to be nervous, I like to tell them that nerves are earned. Nerves mean that you care about things, and not just the results. Nerves mean that you understand the stakes. But if we lean into those nerves instead of trying to deny them, they can become a valuable tool.

Show me a fighter (or any competitor) who isn't nervous before a competition, and I'll show you a fighter who's about to lose. Nerves keep us sharp. They keep us safe. And they're not the bogeyman everyone thinks they are. They're natural and normal and everyone feels them. Your opponent is nervous, too. His coaches are nervous. *Your* coaches are nervous. The referee is nervous. The timekeeper is nervous. Nobody wants to mess up, and if you care about something deeply, the more nervous you should be. And the better you get, the higher the stakes, the more nerves there are to contend with.

If we're playing a friendly game of darts, nobody's all that nervous. But if I throw $100 down and say that the winner gets to keep it, everyone's nerves kick up a notch. Raise that $100 to $1,000 or $10,000, let alone $1,000,000, and people really start to care about the stakes of that game. Now add twenty thousand screaming fans and another two million TV viewers to the mix. Add several dozen reporters and analysts. You know it'll be all over the news the next day whether you win or lose, and that everyone will be judging you. That's a lot of pressure. But it isn't real. Or earned. What's earned is a main event of a UFC pay-per-view in which you're fighting for a title. That takes a lot of time. A lot of fights. A lot of wins. And it means a whole heck of a lot, not only to you but to your family, your coaches, the folks in your hometown. Those nerves aren't given to you. They're not just a present. Everyone in the crowd or watching on TV doesn't have those nerves because they didn't earn them. They *can't* have those nerves. They don't get to have those nerves. But you do. They're yours. You earned those nerves, so wear them proudly. March into the cage with them on your shoulder and look around the crowd. All those people wish they could trade places with you, but they can't. They didn't earn it.

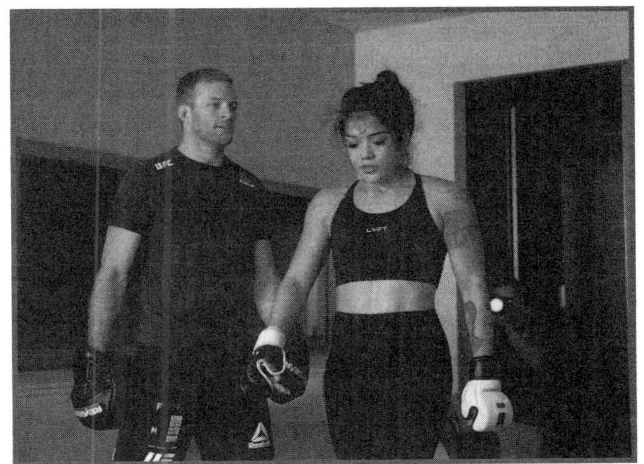

Tracy had imposter syndrome and didn't believe she belonged in the big show.

Seigher Brown

I've trained Tracy Cortez since she was an amateur. She's one of the toughest people I've ever been around, and she holds a special place in my heart, but the truth is that her nerves nearly did her in before her UFC debut in Brazil in 2019.

Tracy had a bit of a rough upbringing and had endured some challenging things in her personal life, but a victory in Dana White's *Contender Series* put her in a position to compete in the UFC. We were in the back of the gym and I don't even know what we were doing there, but I could tell that

Tracy was emotional and upset. I asked her what was bothering her and she said, "I can't do it. The pressure is getting to me. This is all I've ever wanted, and now it's here, and now I'm freaking out. I can't handle all of this." She was having a full-on panic attack. It's not uncommon for people to freak out when they stare at their dreams—when they finally make it to the NFL and the first kickoff takes place. When the first basketball is tipped. When you're shaking hands in the NCAA wrestling finals. Sometimes people let the moment become bigger than it actually is. They can't handle the dream. It's too big. They've made so much out of this moment that they don't realize that what's in front of you is the moment, not getting that close to it. So often, they panic and can't perform. The pressure builds and the pipes burst and the adrenaline floods and they go out with a whimper.

I looked her in the eye and said, "Are you kidding me? This isn't too much for you at all. Look at what you did in the *Contender* series. You mauled that girl, and that was right after the most extreme weight cut I've ever seen in my life" (she lost 19–20 pounds in a 24-hour period).

"You can handle this," I said. "And not only can you handle this, I could put ten thousand times more pressure on you and you will handle that, too. You are one of the most mentally strong people I've ever known in my life. These nerves aren't going to break you. You will show up and you will perform. And you need to understand how strong you are, because I have *seen* how strong you are. I'm not worried about you at all. You're one of the few people I know who will not crack under the pressure. So let's give you *more* pressure. Take *all* the pressure. You're the one who's going to take that last shot at the end of the basketball game. You're the one I'm passing the ball to when the game is on, and you're gonna make that shot."

Tracy paused for a second, looked at me, and said, "I am. I *am* going to make that shot. I can fucking do it." And she did. She went down there. She made weight. And she fought and won her debut in Brazil. Against a Brazilian, no less. And she went five years before finally losing in the UFC.

Success is 90% mental.

STRONG MINDS WIN

We've heard over and over again that sports are 90% mental, and I agree with this statement wholeheartedly. I've said it time and again, I'd take a less-skilled fighter, who doesn't realize he's not as good as he thinks, over a skilled fighter who questions himself, any day of the week—twice on Saturdays (Fight Day!)

SOMETIMES, IGNORANCE *IS* BLISS!

Why is it, then, that athletes (many of whom know how important the mental aspect of a sport can be) train countless hours throughout the week to hone in on their physical, sport-specific skills, but many don't give even a thought to any sort of mental training? So, if a sport is 90% mental, why are we spending 90–100% on physical training and virtually zero time on becoming mentally prepared for an optimal competition mindset? It certainly sounds like a recipe for failure. If an army general knew his enemy was going to strike, knowing the enemy had the most powerful navy in the world, but spent all of his efforts on defending a land raid, we'd all expect that general to fall pretty easily, right? Defeat is imminent. If a teacher gives you a hint of what is going to be on the test—grammar—and you focus on spelling, why would you be surprised when you

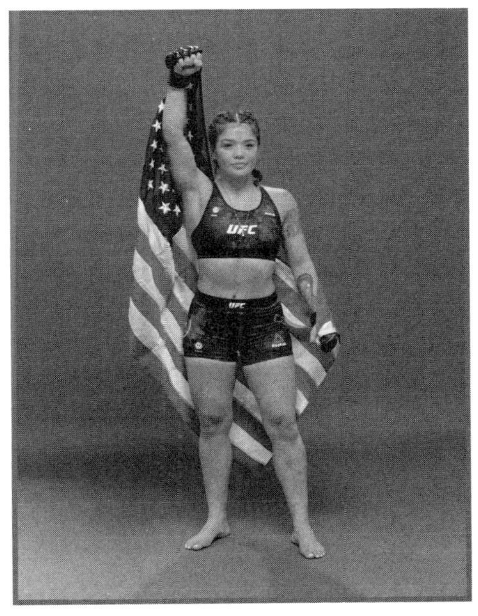

Tracy has always been a mental oak, and I honestly believe it's her best attribute. *Seigher Brown*

failed the test, or, if not failed, certainly didn't perform to the level you knew you were capable of?

We know what we need to do, but we don't do it. We let our mind wander, which can be deadly, in terms of our competition mindset, but we let it do so anyway. We give it a voice, a thought—and we don't need to. We can turn it off, which we should do. We need to turn the volume down, otherwise we find ourselves in self-doubt before competition, and thinking too much mid-fight, which leads us into "analysis paralysis" or the dreaded "adrenaline dump." Both of which are fight, and career, killers.

YOU CAN ONLY CONTROL SO MUCH

> *God, grant me the serenity to accept the things I cannot change,*
> *Courage to change the things I can,*
> *And wisdom to know the difference.*
>
> —Reinhold Niebuhr

Now, hear me out: I'm not religious, but this prayer by the theologian Reinhold Niebuhr is possibly the greatest key to mental strength an athlete, or anyone in the world (athlete or not), could ever have—especially those facing anxiety or any sort of mental adversity.

Years ago, I was a fledgling fighter. I had a record of 11–2 and I held a win over Melvin Guillard, which led, as I mentioned earlier, to me being asked to become a participant on the second season of *The Ultimate Fighter*, where doctors ultimately found a brain aneurysm in my carotid artery. If that wasn't enough, a couple of years later, my wife had a grand mal seizure (the really bad kind) and also had to have brain surgery, though hers was much worse than mine—she needed a craniotomy (a piece of her skull was removed), and then they removed a piece of her temporal lobe.

I'd always been a bit of a mental oak before my brain injury. I loved being the center of attention. I loved talking in front of crowds (even in front of thousands of people), and I wasn't nervous about pretty much anything—certainly not fighting. After mine and my wife's surgery, though, I became emotionally frail. Mentally weak. I developed anxiety in pretty much all facets of my life and became a hypochondriac—I thought any headache, any discomfort, was my brain about to pop. Death was always imminent. But I also developed numerous other fears, including a fear of flying and even social anxiety—I'd begin to sweat uncontrollably and hyperventilate while having normal conversations with friends I'd known for years.

One day, I sat on a plane on my way to visit my oldest sister in New York state. I was sitting in an aisle seat in the back of the plane as I gripped the arm rests tightly—the sweat percolated through my skin, forming drops that leaked down my temples. My chest heaved up and down. My anxiety levels were through the roof. I told myself I was going to die. The plane was going to crash. I would never make it to New York in one piece. What was I doing? I had to get off the plane. I had to get off or I was going to die. I knew it. I knew *THAT*!

But I didn't get off the plane. I sat there, fearing for my life, and I just sat there on the plane, waiting to be flown into my death. And then it happened. I don't know why. I don't know how. My mind was clear. *Clarity*. I thought, "If you really think you're going to die if this plane takes off, then you need to get off right now. And if you don't really think you're going to die, stay on, and accept that the power of this flight is in the pilot's hands, and there's absolutely nothing you can do. If you really think you're going to die, get off the plane!

That's something you can actually control. But after that, you can't control anything, and you need to be okay with that. Trust the pilot, and let him do his job."

And like that!, my palms released from the arm rests, and I was never afraid to fly again. Little by little my anxieties lifted, and I became mentally stronger by the day—all because I realized I was powerless to do anything about the things I cannot control. Being okay with that. But the other side to that is understanding what I can control and DOING SOMETHING ABOUT THAT! There are certain things I can control in my life: how organized I am, how much time I waste, how I treat people, what I eat, whether I stay up too late or drink too much. Those are things I can control, and I need to ensure that I am actually controlling them. If I stay up late and watch an extra episode of *Stranger Things* or drink some beers, I'm going to be tired in the morning—disrupting my entire day. If I procrastinate on getting fighter training schedules built and watching film, I'm going to feel that anxiety over the week, and I won't be mentally calm. If I am rude to my children, they are going to be rude back. The list goes on and on and on. For each thing I can control, but I don't, it creates a little anxiety in my life, or a little uneasiness, or wastes time that I don't have—in short, if I don't control the things I can control, it makes my life more difficult.

Anxiety is created by allowing our brains to obsess on what we can't control, and what the future will hold for us.

LETTING GO OF CONTROL IS LIBERATING

As fighters, we have an endless list of what we can control or not, but it only makes sense to worry about the things we can control. If we spend our time worrying about the things we can't, we waste useful time (which could be spent actually controlling things), but more importantly, we create anxiety. Anxiety is the killer of athletes. Anxiety creates adrenaline dumps. Anxiety has us paralyzed in analysis as someone is punching us. It keeps us up at night. It makes it hard to cut weight (by creating an overload of cortisol, our stress hormone). Anxiety inhibits our body's ability to heal itself.

BUT YOU MUST CONTROL WHAT YOU CAN

We can control how prepared we are for competition. We can control our diet. Our conditioning. Our flexibility. We can game-plan and prepare for an opponent through film and repetitious training. We can control which direction we circle and how well our submission game is. We can control how we set up our kicks and punches and knees. What we can't control is what our opponent does. We can't control whether we get knocked out or not. We can't control if we win or lose. *Wait? What? What do you mean I can't control if I win or lose?* Nope. You can't control that, but there's more to what you can and can't control, and it comes down to the way you frame it. And if you take control of every component of your training, then you are prepared, and that's all you can ever ask for when confronting any challenge—the ability to meet it head-on. Preparation is the grim reaper to nerves.

NERVES ARE NOT THE GOAL

I was in the locker room at Fight Ready as one of our amateur fighters was washing his hands. Class was just beginning. He seemed to be getting ready to leave, as opposed to getting ready to train.

"How's it going?" I asked.

"I'm just trying to get through the day—just trying to stay optimistic, I guess," he replied.

"What does being optimistic have to do with anything? What does that matter at all?"

"I guess I'm just trying to look at things in a positive way since they've been hard lately."

"But what does optimism have to do with anything? When you wake up in the morning and there are dishes in the sink, does it matter if you feel like doing them or not? No. The dishes have to be cleaned, and it doesn't matter if you feel like it or not. When the farmer looks outside in the morning, does it matter if it's raining or if he's happy about the work or whether things could be better? No. He has to get out there and plow the fields whether he's happy or not. Things need to get done, regardless of how we feel. We need to pay our rent and eat, and feelings don't have anything to do with any of it."

I couldn't believe it, but the very next day I was in the sauna, and one of the fighters, Alonso, was sweating in the hot box with me. He had an upcoming fight, and we were discussing his weight, the cut, fight plans, and the lot. He then said something that invoked the same sentiment as the day prior.

"I'm always nervous before the fights. I always think, what am I doing? This is crazy. I'm never doing this again. I wish I was one of the fighters who loved to fight. Who got really excited to fight."

I answered similarly but elaborated further.

"What does being excited have to do with fighting? What does that matter? If you're really happy and excited to go into the fight, but then the third round comes and you're dead tired and getting elbowed in the face—well, you're not excited to be there anymore—so does that mean you just quit? The excitement is over so you're out of there?"

"I guess not," he said.

"Now, on the other side, if you're scared shitless and don't want to go in the cage, you're still going to fight, right?"

"Of course! I would never pull out of a fight," he said in his thick Spanish accent.

"So, your feelings don't matter. Don't let your feelings get in the way of your goals. Children do that—children allow their emotions to dictate their actions. 'I don't feel like brushing my teeth.' 'I don't want to clean my room.' But we're adults. We're competitors. Why are we allowing emotions to dictate our actions? Why let emotions get in the way of your goals?"

One of my other fighters, Ray Waters, always responds the same way when I ask him how he's doing: "Don't matter how I feel. Let's get to work."

I've heard so many sports psychologists and "mental/mind" coaches try to euphemize nerves, downplay the nerves. "Look at the nerves as something fun. Look at the nerves as something positive." I even stated earlier in the chapter that the nerves from fighting or competition are the same as going down a roller coaster. Fear is fear. Nerves are nerves. And they're all the same regardless of the origin of their presence. They do keep us safe, so not only are they needed, but they're a GOOD thing! Now, shifting the mindset from negative to positive is definitely better than the original alternative (nerves being perceived as fear), but there's another alternative we're not talking about. Nobody's talking about it.

Why are we giving our nerves that much power over us to begin with? Why are we giving so much power to an emotion?

Athletes and sports psychologists (and the fraudsters in the mental space) are talking so much about nerves, but why? Why aren't we just accepting them as they are, acknowledging their existence, and moving forward with our pursuit of a goal? And the more we just accept them living within us like *Venom* (the movie), the more comfortable we become with them. And then the more we compete, the more familiar we are with that feeling of discomfort—and it's really the discomfort that's the problem. As humans, we want to be comfortable even if it means we're miserable—we all know that friend who didn't break up with his girlfriend or divorce her husband because it was easier to be miserable than it would be to be uncomfortable with a new house, partner, life, and so on. Runners use the phrase "Embrace the suck" and it's just that—be okay with the uncomfortable. If someone was pinching you, it would hurt, right? But it's not going to kill you. It's not going to cause lifelong damage—it's just uncomfortable. Nerves make us uncomfortable. They're a phobia for no reason. A fear of sunlight or air or anything—it just doesn't make sense.

Henry Cejudo was talking to a group of wrestlers recently and brought up fear and nerves. He said that anytime he had that nervous feeling of not wanting to do something, he knew it meant he HAD to do it. We have to lean into that feeling.

Before Henry defended his UFC belt against TJ Dillashaw in Brooklyn we were watching the fights in the locker room. There was a wild fight on the monitor, and he turned to me, "Coach, can you believe I'm about to go out there and do that? It's crazy."

Henry hated fighting. He didn't like it one bit. But he wanted to be the best at it, and so he was. The only emotion he ever showed was after his hand was raised.

At the end of the day, goals are goals. The thing is the thing. If we allow emotions to dictate our actions, our goals, and our dreams, we'll never get off the nerves treadmill. Stop giving nerves so much attention. Acknowledge them as normal and move on. Just remember, there's no Christmas gift anywhere.

REFRAME HOW YOU LOOK AT THINGS

Dan Henderson has a great right hand. But I can't worry about that right hand if I'm fighting him. He's either going to throw it or he isn't. What I can control is if my left hand is high, which will negate the right hand. It's all perspective. I can't worry about my opponent shooting takedowns on me—I don't have control over that. But I can improve my takedown defense, and ensure I'm confident in my own skills. I can't control whether I win or lose, but if I'm prepared, with good cardio and good technique, and I fight constantly and do all of the things I know I'm capable of (that I can control) and use what I worked on during my training camp: If I fight to the best of my abilities, chances are, I'll come out the winner. And if not, if I fight the best fight I could have ever fought and still lose? Well, then, hats off to my opponent. There's nothing I can do about that. More often than not, I'll win those battles, but if I don't, that's out of my control.

Winning is our optimal goal, but it's not what we should focus on. We need to focus on the details—the "now"—and those add up to a win or a loss. Instead of focusing on the negative version of a scenario, reframe it so that it's a positive version—one you can control the outcome of. Worrying about a knee won't do you good, but making sure you're moving laterally will. Thinking about your opponent's low kick won't help, but ensuring you're checking kicks correctly will. And so on and so on.

When we focus on things we can't control, we add stress to our lives. It might be little by little, but it adds up. A little stress worrying about bills. A little from your opponent's right hand. A little about whether your diet was as good as it could have been.

I recently asked one of my fighters, "If I could tell the future, and told you that you were going to lose your next fight, what would you do when the cage door closes?"

She replied, "Fight."

Exactly.

When the door closes, you're going to fight. It doesn't matter if your opponent is good at this or good at that. Hell, it doesn't even matter if you already know you're going to lose. You're going to fight your ass off. And at the end of the day, it's just a fight. If you're really that worried, don't step in the cage. Get off the airplane. Don't get in front of crowds. Stay at home. Live in fear. Live with anxiety.

Otherwise, just focus on what you can control, and be okay with what you can't. It'll be a lot better that way.

PART TWO

Strength and Conditioning

Strength and conditioning (cardio) are equally important and very much intertwined as they relate to fight readiness. But what do we actually mean by "strength?" Does it refer to how much weight we can push in a given movement, like in a strongman or powerlifting competition? Or does it instead refer to how fast we can move that weight (think athletic, explosive people like football players)? Do we mean muscular endurance (how long we can move weight or how many reps we can move them for—like in rowing)? Or are we instead referring to aerobic capacity? The answer is part "that depends" and part "all of the above."

While overall strength is traditionally considered to be less transferable to success in most sports than speed, power, and cardio are, nothing works in a vacuum, and the body's different systems are all working in harmony with one another when performing optimally. Different body types competing in different sports (or different disciplines within a sport) require strength specific to those body types and sports. One size does not fit all—which is one of the biggest issues with sports strength and conditioning (S&C) coaches and

Instagram fitness gurus alike—which is why the strength training programs I run my athletes through are custom-tailored to meet their specific needs.

My goal for this book isn't so much to tell you what to do—to give you a course of action—but to show you how to create the best course of action for you or your athletes. I want you to understand the differences between various exercises and the different energy systems involved in sports so you can become empowered and not rely on others as much. Understanding the importance of prioritizing baseline strength and baseline cardio before moving toward "functional/sport-specific" exercises should be an art that you, the reader, can accomplish.

But there's one thing I must note before we continue, relevant to both this section and the next, and it's painful, but I'll help you understand it:

Nothing is certain! You are going to read what I write on each subject shortly, and for every tidbit of information I say, you'll be able to Google sixteen articles or studies that both confirm and disprove what I say. Are lengthened partials superior to a sub-range of motion curls? Well, it depends on who you ask. Just as the egg is good or bad for you depending on the year and the study you're reading, everything has its statistics and studies—trying to decipher which study is "right" is as difficult as figuring out the purpose of life.

Should I consume protein/carbs immediately after working out? Probably. There are studies that say doing so is paramount to recovery and being able to perform the following day, but I've read studies that say it's negligible.

My advice: Do what makes sense, and what's simple. If there is a true benefit to consuming a postrecovery shake, and it's as easy as drinking a chalky substance, why not do it? If you have an option of doing something versus not doing something, and it's cheap, easy, and has little to zero side effects or consequences, why not do it? But again, don't overcomplicate things. The 90% rule reigns supreme, and if you're hitting all of the big things, don't stress about the little nuances that may or may not have conflicting literature. But also feel free to play a little trial and error; you are responsible for, inevitably, what you do and what you don't do. What you eat and don't eat. How you train and how you recover. You are the master of your domain, and you are the one who needs to make the ultimate decision on everything.

But remember, if it sounds too good to be true or too weird to just maybe work—it's probably a snake oil pitch, waiting to prey.

7

THE 90% RULE

I love coffee. I have an overpriced, yet very convenient, automatic espresso maker in my kitchen. I choose whatever beans I want to fill it with and then I hit a button. It grinds the beans, brews my espresso in one- or two-shot options, and then discards the grounds in a receptacle bin underneath. I drink two Americanos (each with three shots) before I leave my house. Then on my way into the gym, I stop by Starbucks or a local spot and pick up another cup of light roast. Around 3 PM, I stop and buy another coffee from a shop during my travels. Twice a year or so, I order a peppermint mocha with soy milk—too much milk makes me feel bloated. I drink a lot of coffee. I buy a lot of coffee. I love coffee. Almost every time I'm seen before 3 PM, I have a coffee in my hand.

If you knew the amount of times I've been told, "If you don't buy coffee for a month, at $7 a day, you'll have an extra $140 a month—that's $1680 a year!" or something similar. Wow, a whole $1680 a year?! That may be enough to feed a family in Haiti, but it isn't going to change my life.

We've all heard it. Whether from our mom, aunt, Instagram influencers, or neighbors—*cut the coffee/energy drink/haircut/(insert random small expense here) and look how much you'll save.* But the average rent for a three-bedroom,

2000-sqft. home in my neighborhood is $4500–$8000 a month, and you think $140 a month is going to change my life? Political pundits, for years, complained of "pork spending" in government bills. "They're giving $800,000 to a public university to study shrimp on a treadmill! We can't go on like this!" Yet we are spending trillions on entitlements and defense. There's an elephant in the room, taking up space, but let's point to the mouse in the corner.

DIET COKES AND BIG MACS

I'm going to get rude. I'm going to be stereotypical. But we're all friends here, and we've all stood in line behind the 300-lb. woman who ordered three hamburgers, two fries, a cookie, and a Diet Coke. We've all said in our head, "The Diet Coke is the key, huh?" It's the calories in the soda that're keeping her overweight, not the 1,200 calories in the fries and single burger. It's not the three bowls of cereal for breakfast. It's not the four donuts during the company meeting.

We get caught up with the little things—in the weeds, as they say. They say start small. Small changes are easier. Large changes are difficult. But all the small microdetails don't matter if the large macrolevel concepts aren't being adhered to.

Inversely, if the macro is balanced, the micro is negligible. If the same 300-lb. woman wanted to make a change and lose weight, and drank a regular Coke a day but cut out the burgers and fries, she'd see huge changes in her body composition. If she ate a balanced breakfast, lunch, snack, and dinner, but ate dessert three days a week (or maybe even nightly), she'd lose weight. She'd be in better shape. If you move out of the $8,000-a-month house into a $4,000-a-month house, you could drink double the coffee from Starbucks a month and you wouldn't notice it. Big things matter. Little things . . . well, are the little things.

In sports it's easy to get caught up in the little things. We see fighters throwing battle ropes. We see NFL wide receivers use KT-Tape for physical therapy and see them jump on tiny platforms and then down and around before running routes, and then every high school player in the country is asking their parents for private lessons at "that one place!"

Everyone wants to find the edge, but can't do 50 pushups in a row.

On a technical level, everyone wants to land the superman punch or the flying arm bar, but can't escape mount, can't stay on balance while throwing a punch. We've all seen Odell Beckham Jr. catch the one-handed touchdown, which is great, but most receivers can't run a route. They can barely get open. They can barely catch a ball during practice with two hands and nobody covering them, and they want to practice the OBJ one-handed-catch?!

What nobody sees, though, is the years OBJ ran uncovered routes on a field somewhere with his friend or uncle or mom throwing passes to him. They didn't see him alone juking and sprinting routes and visualizing someone throwing him a pass. They don't see Canelo Álvarez shadowboxing for hours and hours and hours just to get slightly better with his balance as he throws his jab. They just see the taunt and KO. Just as in S&C, they just see the cameras rolling when Tom Brady is being worked on by a very controversial "movement guy." People want to see the weird stuff. They want to see the "out of the box" training because they've seen the rest a thousand times—but it doesn't mean it works, and it doesn't mean it's the 90%—it's just what the cameraman and producers thought would generate better ratings. Remember, TV is fake, kids. The internet is fake, kids. Social media is fake, kids. And there are "gurus" everywhere trying to sell you something.

THE WORK IS THE WORK

If you're an NFL fan, you've seen Jalen Hurts and the Philadelphia Eagles "tush push" their way to numerous first downs and touchdowns. For those who are unfamiliar, that's when Jalen Hurts quarterback-sneaks it and the entire pile seems to plod forward regardless of who, or what, stands before it—pushing anything in its path forward like the blob, seemingly indestructible. So, how is Jalen Hurts able to move forward so frequently? Is it the balance beam exercises and Bosu ball balance parties or is it because he was squatting 500 lb. and benching 275 lb. as a freshman in college while weighing 200 lb.? Are Genady Golovkin, Andre Ward, Oscar De La Hoya, Canelo Álvarez some of the best boxers in the world during their respective careers because they wore sunglasses and hit "neuro-stimulating" lights and worked on their med ball throws or because they ran countless miles a day for conditioning and hit the bag for hours a day? The big stuff is really what the little stuff is made out of—but it develops through years of boring progressions, not shortcuts and fancy training. Roy Jones Jr. has mentioned on numerous occasions about how hard his father made him work—how Saturdays and Sundays were filled with 8-, 10-, and even 12-hour sessions where he would rep the same boring thing again and again and again.

I think you're picking up what I'm putting down.

Everyone wants the "edge" and I get that. But if there is an edge to find, it's for the Tom Bradys who are in their forties trying to find something to give him one extra year. The edge is for the Michael Phelpses of the world trying to win one more gold after an already illustrious career. As of writing this, Russell Wilson and Justin Fields are vying for the starting quarterback position for the Pittsburgh Steelers—two highly competitive, world-class athletes in their respective roles fighting for that number one spot. For that fight, I completely understand if either of them was to look for that tiny extra little thing that might help them get the starting position, even if it were nothing more than placebo. But even with those examples, they're where they are because of the big stuff. They've already dotted every "i" and crossed every "t" they can with the big stuff—THEY get to dabble in some of the little stuff now. And until you are where they are, you should probably just stick to the big stuff because for most athletes—especially high school, or college, or early level pro athletes (pro fighters)—the "edge" isn't real. It's nothing more than a distraction from the real work: hard work. **Remember, the fastest shortcut is hard work.** But it's a lot easier to look for a shortcut to beat the strong guy than it is to become strong. It's a lot easier to cut the Diet Cokes out than it is to eat an overall healthy diet.

Dr. Mike Israetel, a sports science PhD and Brazilian Jiu Jitsu black belt, hates gimmicks and calls them "distractions from foundational movements." In an interview with me for this book he says, "Everything we do in sports has to be looked at in terms of ROI [return on investment]. How much time and energy am I putting into this versus what I'm getting out of it?

"The purpose of strength conditioning is actually very explicit. It is to address the fitness characteristics that are not sufficiently addressed in your MMA training and have a positive ROI when contra-balanced to either more MMA training or doing other strength conditioning things."

THE MAIN THING IS THE MAIN THING

Strength and conditioning should not be the main thing. Unless you are running a race or entered in a powerlifting competition, the sport is an athlete's main goal; S&C is supplemental. We should spend as much time in our sport as possible to gain all the skills as well as the physical strength and conditioning aspects we can. Strength and conditioning's role is for filling our deficiency gaps. If you're constantly losing wrestling matches because you're getting tired in the third period or are getting pushed back from the defensive tackle in your football games because you're not strong enough, that's where S&C comes into play. If you're losing in those areas because of a technical deficiency, maybe

S&C can help you (being more prepared physically never hurts), but maybe there's a sport-training avenue that should be looked at as well.

But most of us are going to have deficiencies in our sport, and getting stronger, faster, and better conditioned are great ways to fill those areas of weakness, and the time we have in a day to physically spend training is limited by our body. We can only spar so much before we get cut or concussed. We can only wrestle so much before we strain a ligament. We can only hit the bag so many times before our shoulders hurt. And so we go to the weight room or the track or the pool.

RETURN ON INVESTMENT

As we just said, there's only so many hours in a day where we can train, so we need to ensure we're making the most out of every single rep and sprint we perform. If we're a general population fitness enthusiast or we just want to look good or live a healthy lifestyle, over or under training doesn't really matter, but for athletes who eat, sleep, and breathe the sport, every minute counts!

So what is our 90%? On a physical level, again, we're not talking superpowers in one area, we don't want to be a savant, we're talking holes in the foundation—we're talking minimum needs to be effective. We can always go way above the minimum, and that's what this book is about, but there's no reason to even talk about increasing your 5.5 second 40-yard time if you can't squat or deadlift your own weight! Let's build the foundation and frame for this house before we start talking brass finishes on the cabinets.

THE BARE MINIMUM

Each sport has its own bare minimum. Hell, each position might have its own bare minimum. Do you think a 125-lb. fighter can lift what a heavyweight fighter will be able to lift? Or do you think a heavyweight fighter will have the

VO_2 max (maximum oxygen consumption during exercise) a 125-lb. fighter will? Absolutely not. And a soccer player doesn't need the strength of a football player, just as a wrestler won't have the vertical jump of a basketball player.

But let's quantify some things because, at the end of the day, we do need data. Sometimes it doesn't mean anything, but sometimes it's nice to know where we compare amongst our peers. I've compiled a list of some 50% markers, 80% markers, and 90% markers for four common sports regularly played at the high school level, collegiate level, and professional level (I'm considering MMA/Olympics as the professional level of wrestling, not WWE). I looked at a few common strength movements (bench press, squat, dead lift), VO_2 max, and a one-mile run time. There are a billion other physical markers I could have used, but these seemed to me to be some of the most common exercises athletes will perform, and all are very accessible (the VO_2 max test is generally performed at a professional facility) to pretty much anyone.

Look at the following charts. There's a huge jump from most high school level numbers to the collegiate numbers, and a jump from collegiate to professional, albeit less so. If you're an average human thinking average human things, falling into the 50th or 75th percentile marks as a high schooler won't make a difference, but if you want to make it to the NCAAs and make the team, you better be eyeing the 90th percentile or above numbers. Why? Well, only about 6–7% of high school athletes compete at the NCAA level. Of college athletes who go pro: about 1.6% of college football players sign to the NFL, and only about 1.2% of college basketball players make a professional roster. And wrestling? We can count on a few hands and feet the numbers who make the Olympic squad or go on to MMA and actually earn enough to support themselves and their families. (A note on the wrestling numbers: these are much less studied and are based on self-reporting at various levels of NCAA wrestling, and vary tremendously due to weight classes.)

WRESTLING

METRIC	LEVEL	50% ILE	80% ILE	90% ILE
Bench Press	High School	135-185	200-225	225-250
	College (D1)	185-250	250-300	300-350
	Professional	225-315	315-365	365+
Squat	High School	225-315	315-365	385-405
	College (D1)	315-405	405-465	465-500
	Professional	405-550	550-650	650+
Deadlift	High School	315-405	405-450	450-500
	College (D1)	405-500	500-600	600-650
	Professional	500-650	650-750	750+
VO_2 Max	High School	45-50	52-55	55-60
	College (D1)	50-55	55-60	60-65
	Professional	55-65	65-70	70+
40-Yard Dash	High School	5.2-5.8	5.0-5.2	4.9-5.0
	College (D1)	4.9-5.4	4.7-4.9	4.6-4.7
	Professional	4.7-5.2	4.6-4.8	4.5-4.6
Mile Run	High School	6:30	6:15	6:00
	College (D1)	6:00	4:45	5:30
	Professional	5:45	5:30	5:15

FOOTBALL

METRIC	LEVEL	50% ILE	80% ILE	90% ILE
Bench Press	High School	175-215	210-250	243-275
	College (D1)	300	345	370
	Professional	315-455	365-475	455-500
Squat	High School	255-295	344-365	385-465
	College (D1)	395	430-455	500
	Professional	465-600	550-650	650-700
Deadlift	High School	370-408	423-500	510-550
	College (D1)	500-550	600-650	700
	Professional	600-700	700-750	750+
VO_2 Max	High School	38.5	45	49
	College (D1)	45	52	55
	Professional	48-55	55-60	60-62
40-Yard Dash	High School	5.0-5.5	4.9-5.0	4.7-4.8
	College (D1)	4.7-5.0	4.6-4.8	4.5-4.6
	Professional	4.4-4.8	4.3-4.5	4.2-4.4
Mile Run	High School	7:00	6:30	6:00
	College (D1)	6:30	6:00	5:45
	Professional	6:00	5:45	5:30

SOCCER

METRIC	LEVEL	50% ILE	80% ILE	90% ILE
Bench Press	High School	95-135	150-175	185-200
	College (D1)	150-225	225-250	250-275
	Professional	175-250	250-300	300+
Squat	High School	135-250	250-300	300-350
	College (D1)	250-350	350-400	400-450
	Professional	300-450	450-550	550+
Deadlift	High School	200-300	350-400	450
	College (D1)	350-450	450-550	550-600
	Professional	450-600	600-700	700+
VO_2 Max	High School	38-45	48-50	55+
	College (D1)	45-55	55-60	60-65
	Professional	55-65	65-70	70+
40-Yard Dash	High School	5.0-5.5	4.9-5.0	4.8-4.9
	College (D1)	4.8-5.2	4.7-4.9	4.6-4.7
	Professional	4.6-5.0	4.5-4.7	4.4-4.5
Mile Run	High School	6:30	6:00	5:45
	College (D1)	6:00	5:45	5:30
	Professional	5:30	5:15	5:00

BASKETBALL

METRIC	LEVEL	50% ILE	80% ILE	90% ILE
Bench Press	High School	95-150	185-200	228-250
	College (D1)	225	250	269
	Professional	250-350	300-375	350+
Squat	High School	195-265	315-350	365-400
	College (D1)	265	305	315
	Professional	365-500	450-550	550+
Deadlift	High School	300-350	400-450	500
	College (D1)	400-500	500-600	600+
	Professional	500-700	650-750	750+
VO_2 Max	High School	40-45	48-50	52-54
	College (D1)	50	55	60
	Professional	55-60	60-65	65+
40-Yard Dash	High School	5.2-5.8	5.0-5.2	4.9-5.0
	College (D1)	4.9-5.4	4.7-5.0	4.6-4.8
	Professional	4.7-5.2	4.6-4.8	4.5-4.6
Mile Run	High School	7:30	7:00	6:45
	College (D1)	6:45	6:30	6:15
	Professional	6:15	6:00	5:45

So what should you shoot for? It all depends on where you're at in your athletic journey. If you're a high school athlete looking to play D-I, you'd better be shooting for the top echelon of 90% or more—especially in sports like football, where numbers (40-yard dash, bench press, squat) mean a lot more than those same numbers do as a college soccer player or wrestler.

If you're currently ranking in the bottom 25% of a lift or run and want to compete at the next level, you better work toward climbing the percentage rankings, but if you're in the NFL, do you need to be in the top tier? Do you need to be in the 95th percentile of bench press or 40-yard dash? No. It definitely couldn't hurt. Let's go back to our Xavier Worthy mention earlier. He recently took the top spot in the NFL combine's 40-yard dash and had an amazing rookie season, but what about the rest? What about all of the other pro bowler and all-pro players that are in the middle of the pack on their weight room numbers, but have the skills to make up for any athletic deficiency? Skills pay the bills, remember that.

But now you know where you should be at. You know what to focus on. And don't get distracted by some shiny new toy on the sidelines or some guru who says he has a trick to give you that competitive advantage others just don't know about. It's a lie, but I bet he sells it at a great price!

8

WHAT DIFFERENCE DOES IT MAKE?

Understanding the differences between strength, power, explosive/dynamic movements, plyometrics, aerobic capacity, anaerobic capacity, VO_2 max, and more importantly what they do and don't do, is critical to getting the most out of one's workouts. Running a marathon at a 10 min/mile pace (aerobic) and Nordic skiing to absolute failure (VO_2 max) require very different functions of one's body, so athletes need to know how to train in a way that is specific to their performance goals. Think the difference between an NFL lineman exploding off the line vs a basketball player dunking. NFL = ballistic; NBA = plyometric. And both are worlds apart from a marathon.

Many people call anything with a jump a "plyometric" and that's just not true. Not all jumping movements are the same. A lineman needs to explode off the line using maximal power, which could be worked on by squatting low and exploding forward as far as he can go. But a basketball player doesn't need that. Have you ever seen LeBron James run toward the hoop and then squat down and load his jump? No! He runs and springs off the floor with minimal contact and maximal height. To imply that the two exercises are similar or that the two athletes need to train the same way is a disservice to all athletes. Understanding the differences between these movements and how to properly execute them is one of the biggest challenges athletes face and one of the biggest problems I see with strength and conditioning "coaches." Too many athletes and coaches are being wowed by Instagram influencers posting wild and crazy workouts and integrating them into their strength and conditioning programs when they probably shouldn't.

WHAT'S IN A NAME?

As a practitioner, and even to a somewhat lesser degree, as a coach, I hate defining . . . well, everything. Putting names and labels to things is like putting Play-Doh in a cookie mold. I understand that we have language to define terms to understand exactly what they are. I get it. Linguistically, I love it. But creatively, I hate it.

I taught college English for a few years. I have an MFA in creative writing. I love words. Using the correct term and definition of a word helps us avoid miscommunications when we're arguing with a loved one or we're trying to debate politics. And I love to use my linguistic prowess to help me win arguments—which usually comes into play if I feel I'm slipping and losing the argument! But in MMA—any facet of the sport—the more detailed we get, the less freedom we have to adapt techniques to our own style without the terms we use to define them getting in our way. If I say attack guillotines (chokes) while your opponent is trying to take you down, a fighter might ask, "arm in guillotines?" "high arm guillotines?" "Walsh chokes?" The details get in the way. The details are too restrictive. The same could be said with a jab while boxing. Are we throwing "up jabs" "45's" "power jabs," etc.? *Just throw a jab and make it land!* The rapper Lil Wayne once said he doesn't like writing his songs down because it's too restrictive. If he writes the words down on paper, he doesn't have the freedom to change them. Writing lyrics down holds his creativity back. He got the idea after hearing that another famed rapper, Jay-Z, didn't write his lyrics down either. I'm very vague with the terms I use, and I don't keep up with the new lingo (so many "moves" are named and renamed with the tiniest change in detail).

But I'm a master of MMA. MMA flows through my veins like music danced through Beethoven's fingers. I know what I need to know, so I can break the rules. There's a saying, in pretty much every niche: Know the rules so you can break them. You have probably noticed my style of writing toggles between "perfectly grammatical and structured" and then I use sentence fragments and odd punctuation at other times. I do that to help me explain myself the way I feel I would sound if I were speaking with someone. My understanding of punctuation and grammar is fantastic—near perfect. I can cheat when I want to because I know what I'm doing. The same goes for MMA. There are hard rules, and there are malleable rules. But, if you really asked me to explain the minute differences between two very similar moves, I most certainly could—maybe I'm just old and lazy? Maybe I just don't feel the need to explain myself, as another highly trained coach on my level would get it. I don't know anything about engineering, but I'm sure if I took a couple college courses, I'd know just enough to annoy some really phenomenal working engineers—and I'd give myself away as a novice in one sentence. What's that saying, "better people think you're a fool by staying quiet than relieve all doubt by opening your mouth"? Something like that.

And now the problem.

How do you know if your coach (or any coach, teacher, influencer) is knowledgeable, and trying to limit restraints and is using the "less is more" strategy, or happens to be truly ignorant or a charlatan? And now what about the opposite? Is the coach using scientific terms and fifty-dollar words to impress you because he doesn't really know the subject matter as well as he says and is disguising his inexperience, or does he just have a passion for his subject?

Well, that's why we define things. And if you're already a PhD in this subject or a world-class sports coach, you can skip every definition in this book but, otherwise, let's define some terms so we know what we're discussing, and so when your S&C coach says let's warm up with some "plyos" you know what that actually means. Now, here's the disclaimer! Just because your coach actually knows these terms and adheres to them, doesn't necessarily make him good. And, just because your coach calls a ballistic movement a "plyo" doesn't necessarily mean he doesn't know what he's doing—maybe he's like me and just doesn't want to have to spend fifteen minutes explaining everything to a novice. But YOU need to understand what these terms are, so YOU can make your own educated judgments on your own training and decipher others' subject knowledge.

Bret Contreras, an author with a PhD in Sports Science, says, "The number one thing athletes are missing is the correct goal and then the proper strategy to reach those goals." That is true for both athletes and coaches. Many don't have the tools to properly reach the correct goals because they don't understand the differences between the body's energy systems that are working at a given moment. Everyone wants the next cool new thing, and it's really hard to stick to a plan because, as Contreras says, "gaining glutes is boring. We're doing hip thrust three times a week and it's boring. We're doing abduction and it's boring. We're doing a lot of the same movement and I'm making them do them over and over, and over." Often the right stuff is the boring stuff, and too many strength and conditioning coaches want to impress instead of keeping it simple, because simple is boring.

We'll break down the "jumping" and "lifting" terms here, and we'll leave the "cardio" and "nutritional" terms for later chapters. This is not exhaustive by any means, but for this book, these are the main concepts I will talk about that you'll need to understand. In terms of defining them, I'll lump them in three extremely broad terms: jumping, lifting, cardio. Cardio will be its own chapter, and we'll combine them all in the Holistic Approach chapter.

JUMPING MOVEMENTS

Plyometric

Definitions: There are a ton of slightly varying definitions of a plyometric, but I like this version the best, from sciencedirect.com: "Plyometric exercises are generally defined as brief, explosive maneuvers that consist of an eccentric muscle contraction followed immediately by a concentric contraction." Now, let's define the definition and add on to it! "An eccentric muscle contraction followed by a concentric [muscle] contraction" is, in laymen's terms, shortening and lengthening a muscle while under force. Think of a bicep curl. The concentric movement is bringing the weight up toward your shoulder (the muscle is shortened), while lowering the weight literally makes your arm (muscle) longer, but you're not dropping the weight, it's controlled. While running (a plyometric movement) your leg lengthens as it extends out in front of you (eccentric) and shortens as it pulls you forward (concentric).

But there's more. And this is the real defining characteristic of a true plyometric: ground contact time. To be a "true" plyo, the ground contact of your body needs to be under .2 seconds. Hurdle bounds, pogo jumps, skipping rope (fast), and running (maybe the truest plyometric ever!) are all "true" plyometrics. Some forms of drop and jump pushups are plyometric in nature (depending on contact time).

Benefits: Speed, the ability to start and stop movements faster, agility (the ability to change directions), jumping, improved tendon and ligament elasticity and strength.

Real-world scenarios: Sprinting, wide receivers juking out defenders on routes, basketball players getting open and dunking, fighters changing directions quickly with footwork and punching—most professional sports are going to have massive use for plyometric movements.

What it's not: Plyos aren't just anything with jumping, throwing, or running. Box jumps, squat jumps, lateral jumps, anything with a jump and hold component wouldn't be considered a plyometric. Most catch and throw movements are not plyometric in nature but rather, ballistic, which we'll discuss shortly.

Training plyometrics

As a coach, I think plyometrics are one of the scariest things for me to see any athlete train because they can be overdone so easily, which can lead to major injuries. I often see coaches using jumps and bounds and a combination of plyos and ballistic movements as a form of conditioning, which is like drinking and driving! Plyos should be performed while fresh, at the start of a workout or as a stand-alone workout, with adequate rest time in between sets. If you think about sprinting in a very simplistic manner, it makes it very easy. The purpose of a plyometric is, really, to become faster or jump higher—I'm using the most simplistic form/reasoning here. In order to jump higher or run faster, you have to jump as high as you can and run as fast as you can—break through the proverbial ceiling. Well, if you sprint 80 yards at 100% effort—we'll say you reached 20 mph—and then jog back and try to do it again, well, you're not remotely recovered well enough to repeat that performance, so you end up fast jogging and only reach 15 mph. YOU'RE NOT HITTING THE CEILING! Rest well enough so you can reach your 100% effort again. Eventually, your max effort goes from 20 mph to 20.1 mph and 20.2 mph and so on and so forth. The second you fade to submaximal effort, you're using a completely different energy system and different muscle groups and you're not going to get faster or jump higher. And if you're not sprinting/jumping at 95% effort or above, you're not gaining speed/dynamic ability, but moving into a conditioning phase. Effort is key, and to exert max effort, you need adequate rest.

But what's the issue, you ask? Well, once your muscles begin to fatigue, and then you're attempting to start and stop and change direction at maximal effort, but with submaximal energy to achieve that goal, injuries occur. I've seen it time and again—an athlete tries to push too many jumps and sprints and max efforts into a single session or day, or train maximal effort daily, and they pull muscles, or far worse, tear a ligament because the supportive muscles assisting in quick, dynamic movements aren't strong enough to keep the body safe and injury free.

In addition to being the most dangerous of all exercises to athletes due to the tendency to overdo them, I personally believe plyometrics are some of the most overhyped exercises strength coaches program for their athletes—except for sprinting, which is horribly underprogrammed. Let me explain. And I should also qualify what I mean by "overhyped" as well. I don't mean they're not important. I should say plyometrics are not as important to an athlete's success in relation to how much emphasis S&C coaches have put them into an athlete's workouts.

The standard train of thought is that plyometrics are very important in sports. Wide receivers are juking and sprinting and jumping. Boxers are juking and bounding off the canvas, using the inertia created to throw fast, devastating punches. Basketball players are jumping through the air. Being "athletic" means having a great plyometric muscular ability. So why do I think they are overprogrammed? Because players can get much of their plyometric work by playing their sport. By drilling their sports. By overexaggerating movements in their sport. Get on the basketball court and move and jump and reach for that rim time and again, and you're getting your plyometric work, but you're also getting your sport skill as well. Running football routes again and again at 80–90% max effort is going to get you faster. It's going to make you a better athlete. Boxing is a plyometric sport. Box, and you're going to get springier while you're boxing. People try to adapt their workouts to the sport too often, instead of just playing the sport!

Now, to sprinting. I almost never see anyone other than football players and track athletes sprinting at 90–100% max effort. I don't get that. I've heard S&C coaches time and again say, "Sprinting isn't directly applicable to fighting or wrestling or . . ." What?! Show me a sprinter who isn't a freak athlete and I'll show you a fat marathon runner. Sprinting is THE ultimate plyometric, and the faster a body moves on the track, the faster it's going to move in any facet of sports. Being a better athlete is the best thing an athlete can do for herself in any sport, and sprinting is just going to help that.

Note on plyometrics: Plyos are great for what they're meant for: running faster and jumping higher. But know what the goal is for plyometrics—on a very simplistic level, stiffening the tendons. Stiff tendons transfer more energy than elastic/weak tendons. The entire purpose of a plyometric is to generate more ground contact force, which creates more energy and propels you forward or upward, depending on your goal. So, when performing plyos, don't try to be "springy" during your "A-skips" and "B-skips" but be rigid and stiff and "hit" the ground—"stomp" the ground. Generate force while hitting the ground. Don't try to "absorb" the fall and shock, but meet them and smash them. That constant "stomping" helps to stiffen the tendons, which is what we want. And, remember, speed is all about ground contact force propelling you forward!

Ballistic movements

If a plyometric is fast and springy, ballistic movements are the powerful older brother. Remember, power equals mass times velocity. Ballistic movements are moving weight, whether body weight, a barbell, or even a weighted medicine ball or sledgehammer, and moving that object as fast as possible. The rise of ballistic training began as coaches and athletes noticed a limitation in the weight room with power movements: deceleration—the need to slow down the object in motion at the end of the range of motion.

You can't really throw a barbell in the air at the gym and let it fly out of your hands and into the squat rack in front of you. Nor is it safe to try to catch a 1rep max clean in the air if you were to throw it over your head. So we naturally slow the weight down toward the end of the range of motion, which limits us by a few percentage points of our actual max effort. The controversy with ballistic movements is we don't really know if throwing a 20-lb. med ball as hard as we can at a wall is any better than pushing 200 lb. on a bench press as fast as we can, even if that means we must take some velocity off the top end. It's certainly safer than trying to catch a barbell at the end of a bench press if we threw it in the air; we know that for sure!

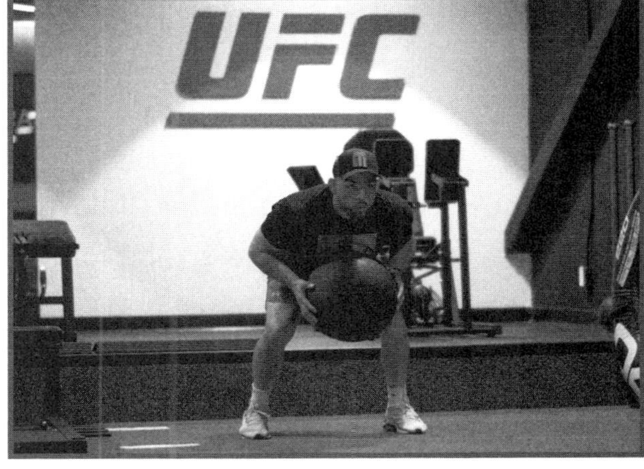

Ballistic movements like throwing heavy things are a great way to build power.

Seigher Brown

What we do know is many people confuse ballistic movements for plyometrics all the time. Frog jumps (loading weight down and leaping forward as far as possible), lateral jumps (pausing after the descent), and many types of box jumps are all forms of ballistic/dynamic movements, but wouldn't be considered a plyometric movement because the ground contact time will exceed the .250 seconds or less needed to be categorized as a true plyometric.

Other forms of ballistic movements are anything where an object is being thrown—sandbags, medicine balls: two-handed med ball throws, one-handed, overhead, med ball slams.

The perceived benefits are high-dynamic movements with greater force. It reminds me of Major League Baseball batters swinging heavy bats before they actually get up to bat—swinging the weighted bat before the lighter bat is perceived to give the batter an easier time when swinging the lighter bat. If I can throw a 20-lb. med ball really hard, I should be able to throw a baseball or a punch even harder. I like the idea of ballistic movements, but I'm not sure I buy the efficacy of them in the throwing sense. What I do like are ballistic-type jumps, such as frog jumps. They can simulate repeated max effort explosive movements similar to a football tackle or block or wrestling double leg, but without the risk of injury of performing those movements live. If you've ever done 10 max effort frog jumps in a row then you know how hard they are, and I love them for increasing VO_2 max (more so than increasing any sort of power).

Here's a quick sidebar: I'm not saying ballistic movements don't help punching power. I'm not saying plyometrics aren't going to make you jump higher. What I'm saying is that when big weight-lifting guys come into the gym they usually hit hard—maybe their cardio sucks, maybe their technique sucks. But big strong people hit hard. People who sprint can run fast and jump high. We can nitpick the details and do all the longitudinal studies we want about how ballistic movements increase (or decrease) throwing power by a few percentage points, but like I said in the last chapter, we only have so much time in the day, we need to make sure we're getting the most out of it. Maybe if we focus on the 90% rule, our need to train plyometrics and ballistic movements might decrease. That said, and here I go talking out of both sides of my mouth again, but if we focus on sprinting (actual max-velocity sprinting), I think you might just get all the plyos you need.

All sports are relative to the application—if your entire sport is the high jump or 100 m dash, you better focus on these. If you're a basketball player . . . MAYBE . . . you should focus on these. Jumping higher and being faster is great, but is it what you need? Maybe you're not making the team because your ball-handling skills suck, or you're 5'7" tall, which has nothing to do with your vertical. I don't know. But you need to really dive into what YOU need, and in wrestling and MMA and probably most sports, plyometrics are PROBABLY overprescribed by the local S&C guru.

Lifting

There are three main types of lifting styles any human is going to implement, let alone an athlete: muscular endurance, power, and strength.

All have their respective benefits, and they have a lot more in common than people might think. They also have a very similar trait with their efficacy—achieving gains in any form really just comes down to effort. You can perform 50 reps of a dead lift and get nothing out of it, or everything out of it. Same goes for 10 reps or 20 or 100 or 2. The number of reps only matters when it's pushing us to max effort and to, or very near, muscular failure. If I perform twelve reps, but I could have hit eighteen, well, I'm probably not going to achieve the gains I'm looking for—and that doesn't matter if I'm training for endurance or power or anything. But if I perform three or three hundred reps, and either of those numbers takes me to where I can't perform a single rep more, well, then I'm going to see gains.

The other major note to grab ahold of while considering lifting is the periodization phase of where you are in your sports cycle—are you out of season, in season, or do you even have a season? We'll discuss periodization more in upcoming chapters, but for now, let's define the different types of lifting.

First, there's a lot of wiggle room for the details of lifting weights. It's like asking, "Are eggs healthy for me?" Well, it depends on what year we're in. As of the writing of this, I'm forty-two years old. Growing up, I remember when eggs were healthy, and then they had too much cholesterol in them, and then the whites were good to eat, but not the yolks. Then the yolks had good cholesterol in them, but not the bad kind. And so on and so forth. I still don't know if eggs are healthy for me or not, but I do love them and probably eat them more than I should—whether healthy or not, too much of anything is probably a bad thing. Just like lifting weights with perfect technique is critical to maximizing gains . . . or is it? Well, it depends on what year it is and what study you're reading. If you have an opinion on any weight lifting concept, there's an article and a study that confirms your belief, and also one that contradicts it. So, let's not get into too many details. Remember, it's the 90% rule that matters. The other 10% is up to each individual to figure out, and we all figure that last 10% out differently. I'm not here to argue if reverse hypers are better than seated hamstring curls. The only people arguing over the minutiae of lifting weights are the scholars and the people trying to sell you why "their way is the best way." When I was growing up, form was everything in the S&C circuit. You didn't bow your back at all on a dead lift or squat—now, even those things are up for debate.

Let's discuss the types of weight training in the order we'll periodize them in an MMA training camp: muscular endurance/base, strength, and then power.

Muscular endurance training

Definition: The ability of a muscle to perform repetitive contractions over an extended period or to stay contracted for an extended period. This is important because not all athletics are speed and power. MMA alone has extended periods where athletes are engaged in long periods of repeated movements (punching) or extended periods where a muscle maintains contraction (think isometric holds) via cage clinching or squeezing a submission for thirty seconds. But we

REP RANGES AND THEIR ROLE IN STRENGTH TRAINING					
TRAINING TYPE	REP RANGE	LOAD (1% OF 1RM)	REST PERIOD	PRIMARY GOAL	EXAMPLE EXERCISES
Muscular Endurance	12-20+ reps	40-60%	30-60 sec	Fatigue resistance	Push-ups, bodyweight squats
Hypertrophy	6-12 reps	65-75%	60-90 sec	Muscle size	Dumbbell presses, leg presses
Maximal Strength	4-6 reps	75-90%	2-5 min	Maximal force	Deadlifts, squats, bench press
Power	1-5 reps	50-70%	2-5 min	Force production rate	Clean and jerk, box jumps

also see muscular endurance and repeated/extended holds play a part in mountain climbing, gymnastics, and other sports.

Muscular endurance characteristics

- **Muscle fibers:** Muscle endurance training stimulates slow twitch (type I) muscle fibers, which are more efficient at using oxygen to generate energy for continuous, extended muscle contractions over a long time. Think "long and slow."
- **Mitochondrial density:** You don't need to know this, but type 1 muscle fibers have larger mitochondria than other fiber types, which

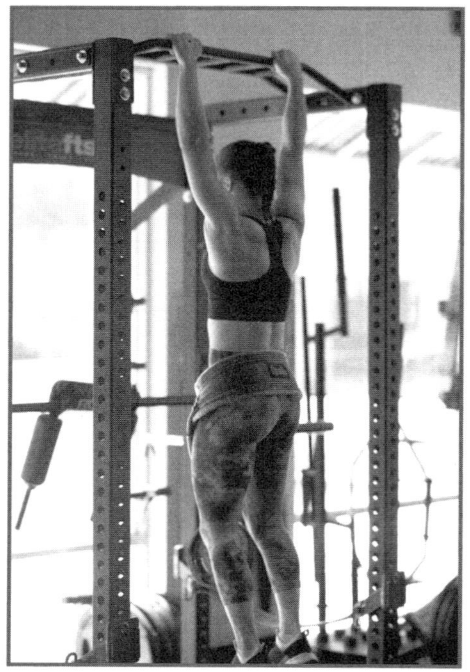

Pull ups or isometric pull ups/ hangs are a great way to strengthen forearms while developing muscular endurance.

Seigher Brown

increases the muscle's capacity to produce energy aerobically.

- **Capillary density:** The capillary is larger, and more dense, which aids in transporting waste out of the cell faster as there's more blood and oxygen able to reach the muscle.

Energy systems utilized

Muscles rely on different energy systems based on the intensity and duration of activity:

Aerobic system

- **Primary role:** Dominant during prolonged, low- to moderate-intensity activities.
- **Fuel sources:** Primarily fats and carbohydrates.
- **By-products:** Carbon dioxide and water, which are easily expelled from the body.

Anaerobic glycolysis

- **Primary role:** Engaged during higher-intensity efforts when the aerobic system cannot meet energy demands.

- **Fuel source:** Carbohydrates (glycogen).

- **By-product:** Lactic acid, which can accumulate and contribute to muscle fatigue.

Generally speaking, people with a greater aerobic base will be able to gain muscular endurance more easily than those who have a lower aerobic base. Muscular endurance is greatly dependent on the aerobic system (oxygen) to fuel muscles and its ability to buffer lactic acid faster through aerobic function.

How to increase muscular endurance

- **Consistent endurance training:** running, cycling, or swimming at moderate intensities over extended periods.

- **High rep weight lifting:** lighter weights and higher repetitions. I like 20–25 reps as the "sweet spot." If you can't hit 20 reps, lighten the load. If you can reach 26, add to the load.

Impact of aerobic capacity and VO_2 max on muscular endurance

- **Aerobic base:** A strong aerobic foundation enhances the efficiency of the cardiovascular system, improving oxygen delivery to muscles and supporting prolonged activity.

- **VO_2 Max:** Represents the maximum rate of oxygen consumption during intense exercise. While a higher VO_2 Max indicates superior aerobic capacity, it is not the sole determinant of muscular endurance.

Sustained endurance activities rely more on the efficiency of the aerobic system and the muscle's ability to utilize oxygen effectively.

Rep ranges

- The norm is 12–20 repetitions per set, but if you're going to go, let's go—and aim for 20–25 reps of lighter weights (40–60% of 1RM [one-rep max]) and shorter rest intervals (30–60 seconds).

To reach failure during muscular endurance training, the body must really go beyond standard failure rates of strength or power training, and failure usually means absolute failure. The amount of fatigue it takes the body to be incapable of performing one push-up after failure is far beyond the fatigue level it takes to bench 300 lb. Imagine grabbing an 8-lb. weight and curling it for so many reps you physically can't lift that 8 lb. one more time—your bicep is dead tired. Now, think of a gallon of milk. It weighs 8 lb., and you are so physically exhausted you can't lift it to pour it in your child's cereal. That is true fatigue! Even after benching 300 lb. to failure, you could still do almost any ordinary task as a human. There are levels to muscular failure!

Example workouts

- **Circuit training:** Multiple exercises performed consecutively with minimal rest (e.g., push-ups, squats, and rows in a sequence) is a very common way of improving muscular endurance. I'm not a huge proponent of circuit training, but during muscular endurance training—I'll allow it.

- Honestly, though, anything you can lift for strength or power, you can lift for muscular endurance as well.

- Don't forget compound movements. Often, people try to focus on individual muscle groups for muscular endurance (biceps, triceps), but I love my athletes to hit their squats, dead lifts, bench presses, and cleans for high reps.

- Diversify your rep ranges. Sometimes hitting weighted lunges for 15 reps of failure is better than hitting unweighted lunges for 50 reps—not always, but you want to be diverse with your muscular endurance—are you a rower or mountain climber? Sometimes you need to hold your entire body weight up for minutes on end as you find the next rock to step on while hanging off a cliff. Other times, muscular endurance is pushing your wheelchair in a 400-m race.

Real-world uses

- **Marathon runners or rowers benefit from muscular endurance training for prolonged activity.**

- Static holds common in mountain climbing, gymnastics, grappling, even polo (riding horses is exhausting!).

STRENGTH TRAINING

Definition: The development of maximal force a muscle can produce against an external object, often over short durations. In English: How much can you

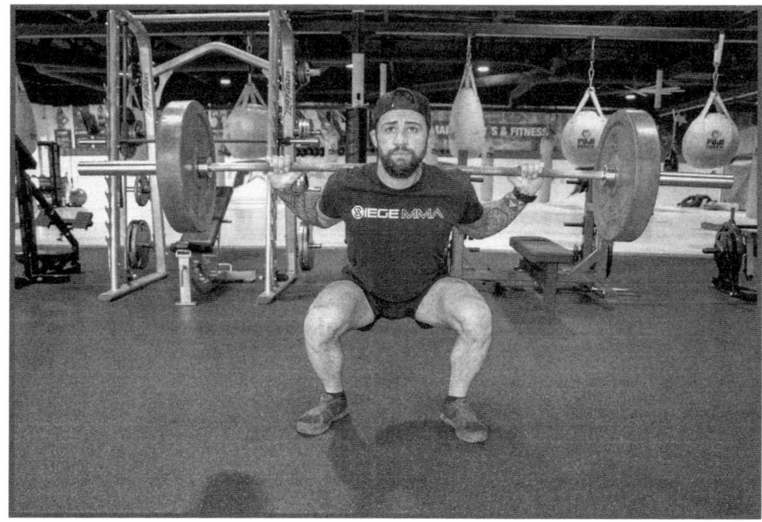

Squats are one of the core-four lifts that should always be in rotation. The others are deadlift, bench press, and cleans (floor or hang). *Seigher Brown*

actually lift? Push? Pull? Speed doesn't matter—we're talking max weights! This is what strongman competitions were made for. Meatheads. And I love it.

Personally, I feel this phase of weight training is the most overlooked part of training in a sports weight room—at least in MMA and combat sports, that is. Utilizing force (power) in athletics is very important. We all know how important cardio is (whether aerobic, VO_2 max, or even muscular endurance). But overall strength is the red-headed stepchild of S&C in athletics. Hell, I even see coaches say how overall strength is "less predictive for sports performance than cardio and power/plyometric activity" all the time. And, to a certain extent, they're right. The issue is that the "minimum standards" aren't being taken into consideration!

There's some fascination for plyometric and power ability in athletics that I just can't understand. "He has a 45-inch vertical!" "He runs a 4.2-second 40!" Both are great. Both aren't going to hurt you as an athlete, but neither will guarantee a win—especially in the UFC or in an Ironman competition. But if a fighter can run that fast or jump that high, great. If not, and even if they have the ability to, let's not forget overall strength and cardio for many sports—especially combat sports like MMA, wrestling, judo, and Brazilian Jiu Jitsu. Let's strength train and cardio train for days and forget most of the rest (if I were limited in my options). Remember, we don't have unlimited time in our lives, and after strength and cardio, we're working our sport—that should give us pretty much all the plyos and power training we'll need.

Strength training and physiology

- **Muscle hypertrophy:** The technical definition is "an increase in the cross-sectional area of muscle fibers, particularly type 2 (fast-twitch) fibers, leading to greater muscle mass and strength," but in English this means the breaking down and rebuilding of muscle fibers, which, if continued over a period of time, results in more muscle fibers and mass (bigger muscles) and (stronger muscles).

- **Neuromuscular adaptations**: Enhanced motor unit recruitment and synchronization, resulting in improved force production. If you've ever gone for a personal record (PR) on a squat or a dead lift, you know how much strain is placed on your nervous system during these excruciatingly long (5-, 8-, 12-second) lifts, and afterward, you're shot. Physically, hours later, you feel like you can barely stand. If you were to try to PR again a few days later—when your muscles might be fully recovered—you can't come close to reaching that PR again. You might need weeks before you feel you can try for it again. That's because your nervous system got hit hard. People don't realize that the nervous system plays a huge role in strength training and athletics. Maximal exertion/effort can sometimes send your body into chaos. It's why I regularly see fighters get sick after their fights—their bodies are shot. They need to be neuromuscularly charged and ready.

- **Connective tissue strength**: Strengthening of tendons and ligaments, which supports increased loads and reduces injury risk. Another highly undermentioned component of strength training is the strengthening of ligaments and tendons. I've seen too many connective tissue tears resulting in surgery to count, and it's about time coaches start preaching the benefits of durability as much as they do strength and conditioning.

- **Bone density**: Increased bone mineral density, contributing to skeletal robustness and a decreased risk of fractures.

Energy systems utilized in strength training

- **Primary system:** The phosphagen system (ATP-PCr), which provides immediate energy for short-duration, high-intensity activities. Phosphocreatine (PCr) replenishes ATP during short, intense efforts. ATP, or adenosine triphosphate, is technically a neurotransmitter that sends signals between cells. ATP is made from glucose during the process of glycolysis, within the mitochondria of the cell, and can be created and delivered via anaerobic or aerobic exercise. Feel smarter yet?

- **Secondary system:** Anaerobic glycolysis, which contributes energy during longer sets or higher-repetition ranges. Carbs, whether simple or complex, will break down quickly by anaerobic glycolysis, giving fast energy to the muscles for use.

ATP is the initial energy source, which will generally support you for your first few reps, but as you start to feel the "burn" you are tapping into your anaerobic glycolysis phase, which burns glycogen and spits out its by-product, lactic acid—which is the "burn" you're feeling in your muscles as it builds up. After stopping the set, an efficient aerobic system buffers (removes) the lactic acid from the muscles, which then allows you to perform more reps. In short, the ATP is the energy for the first few reps. Glycogen is the energy for subsequent reps. And the lactic acid buildup is what eventually stops you from lifting more.

Methods to increase muscular strength

- **Progressive overload:** Gradually increasing the weight, frequency, or number of repetitions in training to challenge the muscles. This is the holy grail of all sports performance! Adding volume, weight, intensity—anything!—gradually over time. Generally, trying to push past 5% a week is going to be difficult as you become more and more seasoned as a lifter. Baby-step it. Inch it. Little by little, you'll get stronger, but if you try to push too much too soon, injury or overtraining may rear its ugly head.

- **Periodization**: Systematic variation of training parameters to optimize performance and recovery. You may want to spend some time targeting one muscle group for a personal record or goal. During that time, other muscles should be on a "maintenance" mode. Or you may decide to do various rest times. Mix in cluster sets. Add circuits. Then mix it up again for a period of time (usually 4–8 weeks).

- **Compound movements**: Exercises that engage multiple muscle groups, such as squats, dead lifts, and bench presses. Training a specific muscle group is absolutely fine, but there's a time dilemma in athletics, and you need the most "bang for your buck" so to speak. I'm not sure the time expenditure toward an individual muscle is going to give adequate ROI. Maybe calf raises—because they are so underworked in the weight room and adding them into a program can really help overall stability, ankle support, and help in avoiding Achilles issues. If you are a bodybuilder or power lifter, isolate to your heart's desire, but as an athlete, choose wisely.

Impact of other energy systems on strength training

- **Aerobic system**: While not the primary energy source during strength training, a well-developed aerobic system aids in recovery between sets and sessions by facilitating efficient removal of metabolic by-products.

Having a more efficient aerobic system assists in clearing out metabolic waste created by muscle use. In other words, after periods of muscle use, and subsequent fatigue, having a stronger aerobic system helps you recover faster, so you can repeat the process.

- **Anaerobic threshold:** Improving the anaerobic threshold can delay fatigue during high-intensity efforts, allowing for more effective training sessions. It may not be a strength issue, but a lactic acid issue. You're trying to hit 10 reps of a lift, but the burn is just too much. Maybe lightening the load for a few weeks and hitting high reps to increase the body's ability to buffer lactic acid is the answer?

Rep ranges

- **4–6 repetitions per set. Velocity isn't a concern with strength training.**
- Heavier weights (75–90% of 1RM).
- Longer rest intervals (2–5 minutes).

Training focus

- **Increasing neural efficiency: recruitment of motor units and synchronization.**
- Hypertrophy of fast-twitch and slow-twitch muscle fibers.
- Structural adaptation: Tendons and ligaments become stronger.

Example workouts

- **Barbell lifts: deadlifts, squats, bench presses, sled pulls/pushes, farmer carries, and overhead presses.**

- Progressive overload: gradually adding weight and/or reps to each lift.

Real-world example

- **Olympic weightlifters focusing on maximal strength to lift heavy loads.**

- Offensive linemen holding off the attacks of defensive ends and linebackers.

I wanted to explain as much as possible of what strength training encompasses before I continue my rant on why I feel it's one of the most overlooked components of athletic trainers: Power is very tiring. It's very inefficient on an energy-expenditure basis. I've seen so many fighters blast double their opponent off their feet in round one, only to be so exhausted afterward they can barely move and end up losing to the way less athletic, way less powerful, way less dynamic fighter.

Going back to Kamuela Kirk, or Ray Waters, a Division I wrestler who could blast double a school bus off the road—they get too tired using that much energy. Everyone would, but the rest of us don't have those superpowers (explosive muscle fibers), so we must use technique and strength to get by. And, let me tell you, it's a lot easier to get stronger through weight lifting than it is to dunk a basketball or sprint at a world-class speed. If these fighters were physically stronger (and had better technique), they wouldn't be so reliant upon their dynamic movements, which are great for football, when you have five- to thirty-second breaks between plays. Just as I mentioned earlier, you don't need to jump the highest or be the fastest or strongest to be the best, you just need to have the minimum physical requirements. I'd much rather be strong in a 15-minute MMA fight than dynamic because that dynamic superpower (along with speed) is usually the first thing to fade away, and then what? Ever notice those guys with round-one KO power (Anthony Rumble Johnson, Vitor Belfort, Conor McGregor, Yoel Romero, Mike Tyson) tend to fade hard and often lose if the fight goes on for a few rounds?

If you are a bit stronger, with a little better cardio, it's going to take you farther (in MMA) than if you can dunk and run a 4.4 forty.

POWER

Power and strength training are very similar, and in most sports, power is going to be the holy grail of lifting. And for many reasons, it should be. The main difference between power lifting and strength lifting is velocity. Similar to the difference between ballistic movement and plyometric, the difference from power to strength is seemingly subtle. Little details; big difference. The simple definition of power is to exert force rapidly with a combination of strength and speed. In weight lifting, power is most synonymous with force from science class; force = mass × velocity. The more mass, the more speed, the greater the force. The difference between a squat of 500 lb. that took eight seconds to lift (we'll call that 3 mph) vs a 350-lb. squat lifted in three seconds (we'll call that 7 mph) is a lot of force. Simple math tells us the 500-lb. squat times three created 1500 lb. of force, whereas the 350-lb. squat times seven miles per hour created 2450 lb. of force. Now you understand why a 280-lb. defensive end who runs a 5.0 forty-yard dash is going to get drafted much higher than someone of the same weight who runs a 6.0 forty-yard dash.

If power is the goal, you need to be in the weight room moving heavy things fast. Squats, dead lifts, power cleans, clean and jerks. Think lifting things from the floor to the ceiling. If that's the trajectory, your weight is headed in the right direction. Many of the exercises used for strength are going to be the same ones used in power (bench, dead lift, squat), but the velocity of the movement will change, and usually the weight will be lower than for pure strength training.

There are different thoughts on the speed of power training, but you don't need to be scientific. Give a good ol "one one-thousand, two one thousand," on the concentric phase (the lifting part) count. If the weight is moving about that fast, you're in a decent range of speed for power. Once the movement starts to slow, rack the weight. It doesn't matter if one rep was performed or eight reps were performed, but when the speed slows, there's more time under tension and your muscles are adapting for a strength movement. Dr. Mike Israetel uses a somewhat crude, but very understandable analogy for this, "You don't need an equation to know if you're sexually aroused. You just know it. The same goes for effort or speed or whatever: you know when you're giving it your all." And you do. You know when the bar is moving fast versus slow. There are countless machines out there that measure the speed at which the bar is moved, and those are great for some teams and coaches, and especially scholars and scientists who are trying to study the exact outcomes of exercises. We want those studies! We need that information on a macro level of sports science. But you, the individual, you don't necessarily need that. And so often adding gadgets takes away from what we already know. It adds steps and complexities to something that should be as effortless as possible—remove the roadblocks. I can't tell you how many athletes I see lose motivation because they left their heart monitor at home and can't track their run or workout.

So how do we lift for power? Strength coach Matt Wiedemer, who's worked extensively with Jon Jones and Henry Cejudo in MMA and countless NFL athletes, broke it down to me in such a great way.

Benefits: Power equals force. Force means you're going to be able to move another able-bodied human when speed is a factor—pulling a semi in a strong-man contest is great, but it won't necessarily help you on the gridiron because of the speed of the movement. Power also has a very beneficial component to athletics—less atrophy. Lifting for power vs lifting for strength will generate less time under tension, and will therefore generate less atrophy (the body's natural breaking down and rebuilding process for muscle synthesis). Being a sore athlete is horrible. Delayed onset muscle soreness (DOMS) is a nightmare when you're trying to run routes or shoot for takedowns.

Real-world scenarios: Go watch *Sports Center* during NFL season, and you'll see what true power is. Guys getting tackled and breaking in two. Go watch old UFC footage of Brock Lesnar blast doubling other NCAA wrestling All-Americans across the cage. Or watch Sammy Sosa blast baseballs into the parking lot.

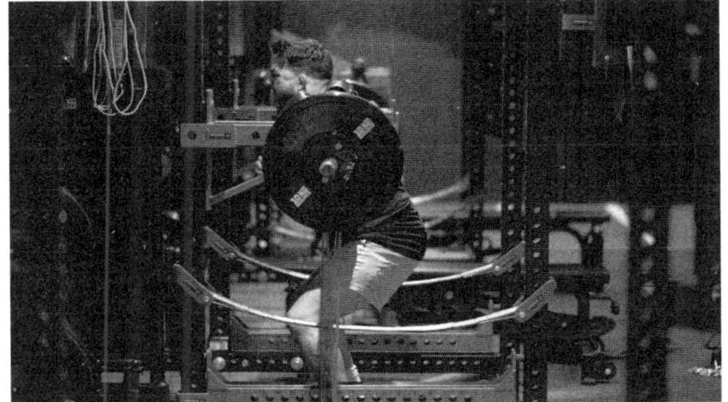

Adding bands to the bar is a great way to ensure athletes are creating as much velocity as possible throughout the entire movement.

Seigher Brown

What it's not: Power isn't ballistic training. Ballistic training is a form of power training, but true power training is moving heavy weights in the weight room. Squats, dead lifts,

Power training

Definition

- **The ability to exert force rapidly, combining strength and speed. Mass × velocity = power/force.**

Rep ranges

- **1–5 repetitions per set.**
- Moderate to heavy loads (50–70% of 1RM).
- Explosive movement focus.
- Longer rest intervals (2–5 minutes).

Training focus

- **Optimizing the rate of force production (how quickly muscles generate force).**
- Activating fast-twitch muscle fibers.
- Improving athletic performance in activities requiring speed and explosive power.

Example workouts

- **Olympic lifts: clean and jerk, snatch, floor and hang cleans.**

- Ballistic training: box jumps, broad jumps, and medicine ball throws.

- Speed squats or dynamic bench presses with resistance bands. Bands are one of, if not THE best way to increase power in the weight room. Matt Wiedemer gave me the best explanation of band training there could possibly be. He said (as I mentioned before about deceleration), "The issue with power training is the deceleration phase needed once our bodies push through the first half of the movement. Ever notice how hard a squat is from the bottom to about a 90-degree angle? Then it's easy. Using lighter weight than your strength training work, but adding a band forces you to drive all the way to the top of the movement, and it becomes hardest at full range due to the band being stretched." Bands force you to "explode" through your entire movement or you're not going to get to the full range of motion, and they remove the risk of throwing an object into the air, while the deceleration problem disappears. Bands, folks!

Real-world example

- Defensive linemen are powerful. Linebackers are powerful. Rugby players are powerful. Mike Tyson was knocking people out with power. Usain Bolt, though probably nowhere near as physically strong as those just mentioned, generates a massive amount of power

DIFFERENCES IN TRAINING TYPES			
ASPECTS	MUSCULAR ENDURANCE	STRENGTH TRAINING	POWER TRAINING
Goal	Sustain force over time	Maximal force production	Explosive force application
Intensity	Low to moderate	High	Moderate to high
Speed of movement	Controlled	Slow and controlled	Fast and explosive
Fuel Source	Aerobic / anaerobic mix	Primarily anaerobic	Anaerobic
Muscle Fiber Focus	Slow-twitch	Mixed fibers	Fast-twitch

through speed—remember, speed AND mass create power. Not just one or the other.

Note on rep ranges and various heart rate zones: Remember, the body is a lot smarter than us and it's predisposed to its genetic foundation, which will smash through any preconceived notions we have as intellectuals.

Some of the rep ranges blend. If you think by sticking to three reps you're only going to build power and avoid any hypertrophy or muscular endurance, you're wrong. Same goes for all the other "reps and ranges." They are going to blend. There's no perfect fine line where one energy system begins and one ends. The same goes for aerobic and VO_2 max cardio. Just because you decide to run at a specific heart rate doesn't mean you will only be in one zone versus another. Again, those lines blur just as the rep lines blur, and you may enter and exit numerous energy systems throughout a workout—even if it's tailored for a specific response/adaptation.

And then there's the genetic factor to contend with.

You could train yourself or an athlete in one range or another and nothing makes sense. Athlete A gets big and strong and fast and lean and perfect with a specific exercise/rep range/HR (heart rate) zone, while Athlete B gets worse in every single area with the same programming.

It doesn't make sense, but the body does what the body does. Finding the right code that unlocks the perfect genetic lock for the individual athlete is a different combination for everyone.

We're dealing with more art and witchcraft than science.

9

ENDURANCE

What are you willing to endure to achieve the goals you've set out to accomplish? In fighting and in life, endurance is critical, and as a trainer I'll be damned if one of my fighters is going to run out of gas before his or her opponent does.

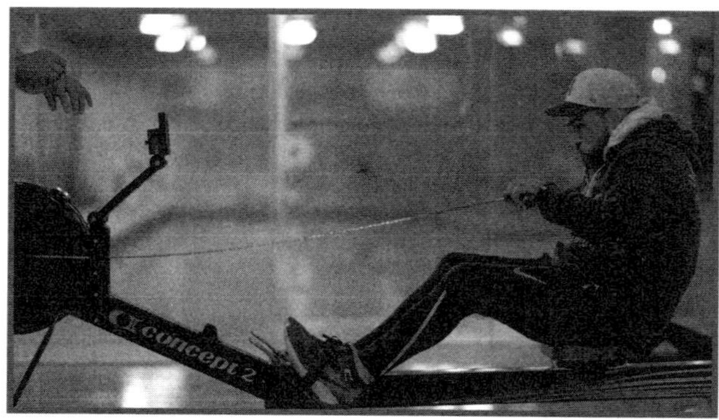

Endurance is probably the most physical component of most sports. Doesn't matter if that's muscular or aerobic. Pushing longer than your opponent is a great way to ensure victory. *Seigher Brown*

One example that almost any avid runner can relate to is the "run slow to run fast" maxim. This might sound counterintuitive to you if you don't run, but when examined a bit closer, it makes perfect sense. An untrained runner might think that the way to achieve a better time in, say, a 5-mile run is to run a distance, whether 1 mile or 5, as fast as one can, then wait a day or two and try again until one's time improves. But there's a few things wrong with that. First, the delayed onset muscle soreness (DOMS) is real. You're going to be very sore, and your muscles probably won't recover for a week, and you will need too many days rest in between workouts. So you reverse-engineer the situation. First, you run your distance . . . slowly. Your heart rate should stay in the aerobic zone (130–150 beats per minute for most). Initially, the 5 miles is at a 12-minute-an-hour pace, while your heart rate is at 130–150 bpm. You won't feel dead afterward, which will enable you to do the same thing within a day or two. Rinse and repeat. And over time that same 5-mile distance, at a similar heart rate and effort level, is run in less and less time as your body becomes more efficient with its aerobic energy system. Your 12-minute mile decreases to 11, 10, 9, etc. and eventually you're running 5 miles in 25 minutes.

But aerobic cardio is only one portion of endurance. There's VO_2 max, which is how hard you can push maximum effort before complete failure—think the last mile or half mile of a race. You're going as hard as you can, and not only are you racing to the finish line, but there's also an internal race to reach that finish line before you just collapse. Muscular endurance—how many times and for how long can you move weight before the burn is just too much? Competitive rowers, climbers, and wrestlers go through this all the time. Their lungs are there. They aren't out of breath, but the muscle burn wins. They need a break for their muscles to buffer the lactic acid. We're not talking maximal weight here, we're talking 30–60% of their body weight, again and again and again. Mental/neural endurance—how long can you focus before you're distracted? And then there's the physical and mental grit to push through it all when the going gets tough!

We previously spoke of muscular endurance training, so I'll stick to the actual "cardio" training in this chapter.

MY MUSE

This section is really my muse for writing this book—it started as a diet book—me wanting to show regular people (civilians) how fighters make weight—how the number on the scale is only for a moment and a farce, which we'll get into later. But the moment the book was expanded to anything other than an extreme weight cutting book, my disdain for MMA S&C coaches took over due to how ridiculously they all seem to approach cardio.

For a moment, we're going to use "cardio" as a general fitness term for "a fighter becoming fatigued or not during a fight," which seemed to be how S&C coaches always approached it—as an individual factor as opposed to a holistic approach that combined numerous energy systems (strength training, zone aerobic training, VO_2 max, etc.).

Again, I'll use Kamuela as the example, as he was one of my first fighters where I wasn't seeing cardio gains through the employment of various strength and conditioning coaches. He's one of the fighters I've mentioned who is very dynamic. Very explosive. He could knock out a bull. I've seen him take down NCAA Division I wrestling champions with his blast double—just by generating enough force. I can't comprehend that dynamic ability with my "bag of milk" athleticism and my body type.

Kamuela got tired during fights. He'd swing hard and wrestle hard and always get the takedown, and if he didn't finish them in round one by knock out or submission, he lost a decision due to fatiguing and losing rounds two and three. Every strength coach said something similar, something along the lines of, "We need to push your lactate threshold. Push you to failure. Rest. And repeat." That's where the circuits came in (and my disdain for circuit training). They all created some sort of muscular endurance exercise mixed with some sort of aerodyne bike and sled push or pull and gave a rest and then repeated it. It never worked. Not for Kamuela. Not for Ray Waters. Not for Hunter

Azure. Not for anyone who had cardio problems and wasn't already a cardio machine. It seems like if an athlete has the energy system and physiology that happens to respond to whatever program the coaches implement, great. If not, they don't seem to have an alternative.

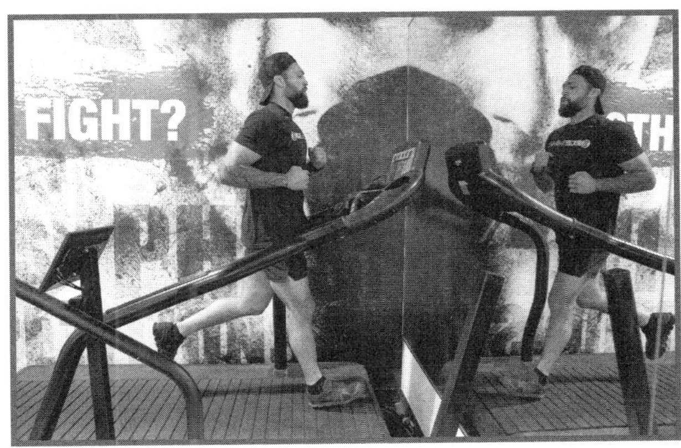

Understanding why you're in a specific heart rate zone is paramount to getting the most out of a workout. *Seigher Brown*

I'm going to discuss how all this fits in more in the upcoming chapters, but the real key to Kamuela's cardio was separating the workouts, where everyone else tried to combine them. My thought process is to train the energy systems (whether strength or cardio) separately, and let the body adapt through skills/sport training, instead of trying to adapt the S&C program for the sport—what some call "sport-specific" exercises, which I don't believe exist. The real key: zone 2 cardio. That's right, zone 2. Light, long, boring runs. Everyone else was trying to redline him to the ends of the earth—push him to absolute fatigue, have him recover, and then repeat the process. It never worked. All it accomplished was to have Kamuela in a state of constant overtraining, which led to injury, illness, and staph infections.

GARBAGE HEART RATE ZONES

I don't know much. And I certainly don't claim to be smart. I'm not a classically trained strength and conditioning coach. I don't have a PhD in the field, nor do I claim to have one. I'm just a simple man who tries to be pragmatic when analyzing concepts I'm unfamiliar with.

I spoke earlier of the "run slow to run fast" mantra. While trying to increase cardio for running, you want to control for two (of the three) variables: heart rate and distance. The third being speed/mph. The more important one being heart rate. If I want to get faster with my 5-mile run time, I don't run 1 mile, 3 miles, or 5 miles as fast as I can. I'll spend too much time burning glycogen. My heart rate will spend too much time in zone 3 and 4. The next day, I'll be sore and feel fatigued. But if I stay in my zone 3 heart rate for the whole 5 miles, I won't be sore, and I can repeat the run the next day or the day after and do it again and again. The key to zone 3 is training the body to burn fat as an energy system, as opposed to glycogen. The moment I begin to go too fast—when I can't really hold a conversation well—I'm burning carbohydrates as fuel. During competition, I want to save those for my dynamic movements. If I'm fighting, I need to explode into a flurry of punches or blast a takedown. Those are going to shoot my heart rate through the roof. They're going to use ATP—broken down from glycogen—as an energy source. But then it will take my body time to replenish those ATP stores. It will take my body time to buffer the lactic acid from my muscles. It will take my body time to lower my heart rate—all while my aerobic system, which is burning fats, is helping my heart rate recover, buffering the lactic acid, and using fat as an energy system so my other systems have time to replenish.

The first time I run that 5 miles, I may be running at a 13 min/mile pace, but if I keep my heart rate at 155 bpm (say that's my zone 2, which depends on my VO_2 max, which can be tested) and I maintain the same distance of a run, my 13 min/mile will eventually fall to 12.5 min, and then to 12 min and then 10, and 9, and 8 min/miles. Eventually, I will be running 5- or 6-minute miles. This concept made sense to me in MMA, and when I heard an interview with Dr. Peter Attia—famed health doctor and podcaster—my ideas were somewhat substantiated, and my interest in trying to help Kamuela with his cardio issues was further piqued. See, Dr. Attia says, "Your overall cardio is like a pyramid. The pyramid can only get as tall as its base will allow for. Your zone 2 aerobic cardio is your base. And the wider it gets, the more height it can support. So if your zone 2 is the base, your VO_2 max effort pushes are the height." You need the VO_2 max pushes to continually break through your cardio ceiling, which is what all the strength and conditioning coaches were pushing Kamuela toward every session, but he didn't have the zone 2 base to support the height of his cardio pyramid!

Cardio, for MMA at least, should only be intentionally performed at two levels: zone 2 and max effort push-till-you-collapse VO_2 max pushes. Anything else is garbage. Now that doesn't mean we won't train within those zones. It just means we won't intentionally train in those zones. Those zones are strictly to be trained at during skills work. During sports work. While we perform cardio, whether zone 2 or VO_2 max efforts, we can control our heart rate. But when we're drilling takedowns, when we're hitting the bag, when we're sparring, we can't just stop or speed up to accommodate for our desired heart rate. The workload is the workload, and we just train in that zone. While playing basketball, you're just playing. While running routes in football, you're just playing. Sometimes it's easy, sometimes it's difficult. It is what it is. You need to focus on zone 2 and VO_2 max. All the other work is done in skills training and sport-specific work. You don't get to dictate that. Anything intentional outside those two zones is just garbage, and there's no reason to try to operate in any of it—that's why circuits are garbage. That's why trying to mimic a fight is pointless while programming for heart rate zones. If you want to simulate a fight, spar. Train. Fight. Your heart rate is your heart rate. And track it. Use a monitor to recover to a desired heart rate and then continue, which is great for lowering heart rate times and recovering faster. But don't try to stay within heart rate parameters while doing so—unless you're trying to push hard through the VO_2 ceiling or are using light skills work for zone 2—which we'll discuss shortly.

I don't mean to be dismissive, but we don't know how our body is going to physiologically respond to certain stimuli. If we try to mimic a fight or a football game or a wrestling match, we don't know if what we're programming is actually doing what we want it to. Our bodies go in and out of zones and energy systems seamlessly while we exercise and play sports. I really love to have the athletes work hard for certain times and light for others and lift for strength or endurance or power separately and let the body put it together. We think we know. But what we do know is how to get strong. We know how to increase VO_2 max. We know that zone 2 cardio increases the mitochondria in cells, which allows for us to convert glycogen into ATP and use it. We don't know if our "sport-specific circuits" are doing the same. And what of adrenaline? What about nerves? What about psychology? All of those factor in somehow, and we don't know how. Keeping it as simple as possible and playing our sport more allows for all the "functional" adaptations we need.

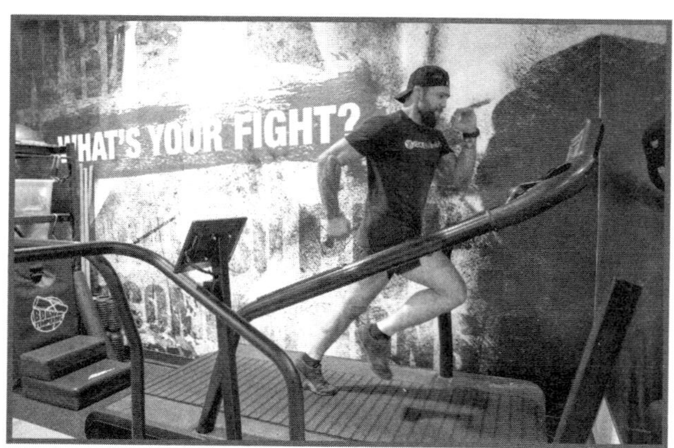

Hard treadmill sprints for 10–30 seconds with long rest periods in between are a great way to push your VO_2 ceiling. *Seigher Brown*

For informational purposes, I want to discuss the main heart rate zones, even if I don't recommend you use them for MMA because I want anyone to be able to adapt any component of this book to their sport, whether MMA or water polo. Knowledge is power, and I want to give you the power to think for yourself. I've spent too much of my athletic endeavors assuming, or hoping, others knew what they were talking about . . . just to be let down.

Heart rate zones and their role in VO_2 max and aerobic cardio

Heart rate zones are ranges generally expressed as a percentage of your maximal heart rate. The simple version is to use 220 minus your age, and then you get your max heart rate. But, as an athlete, that's nonsensical. Go spend a couple hundred dollars on a VO_2 max test, and then you'll know exactly what your VO_2 max is. Take the guesswork out of the equation.

Zone 1: recovery (50–60% of MHR)

- **Description: Light, easy effort; conversational pace.**
- **Physiology**:
  - Relies almost exclusively on fat as a fuel source.
  - Improves circulation and aids in active recovery.
- **Training goal**: Recover between intense sessions, build a base.
- **Example**: A brisk walk or easy cycling for 30 minutes.

Zone 1 is great for active recovery. Go for a walk. See nature. Walk around the mall—if you're over 65, otherwise you're just going to look weird.

Zone 2: aerobic base (60–70% of MHR)

- **Description: Moderate effort; can hold a conversation comfortably.**

- **Physiology**:
  - Enhances fat metabolism and mitochondrial density.
  - Increases capillary density for oxygen delivery.

- **Training goal**: Build endurance, improve metabolic efficiency.

- **Example**: Long, slow distance runs or bike rides.

THE GOLD STANDARD IN AEROBIC TRAINING!

Zone 3: aerobic threshold (70–80% of MHR)

- **Description: Challenging yet sustainable effort; conversation becomes difficult.**

- **Physiology**:
  - Uses a mix of fat and glycogen as fuel.
  - Improves cardiac output and stroke volume.

- **Training goal**: Transition zone; builds endurance and speed.

- **Example**: Tempo runs or moderate cycling for 20–30 minutes.

Zone 4: lactate threshold (80–90% of MHR)

- **Description: Hard effort; cannot sustain for long without fatigue.**

- **Physiology**:
  - The body begins to accumulate lactate faster than it can clear it.
  - High reliance on glycogen as a fuel source.

- **Training goal**: Improve speed endurance and lactate clearance.

- **Example**: 20-minute intervals at race pace with rest in between.

Zone 5: VO_2 max zone (90–100% of MHR)

- **Description: Maximum effort; unsustainable beyond a few minutes.**

- **Physiology**:
  - Requires maximum oxygen uptake.
  - Primarily anaerobic; heavily reliant on glycogen and creatine phosphate.

- **Training goal**: Increase VO_2 Max, improve anaerobic capacity.

- **Example**: 3–5 minute sprint intervals with equal rest.

MY FAVORITE EXERCISE ON THE PLANET IS 400 M SPRINTS FOR THIS. THEY WILL CHANGE YOUR LIFE.

KEY DIFFERENCES BETWEEN VO_2 MAX AND AEROBIC CARDIO		
Aspect	**VO_2 max**	**Aerobic cardio**
Focus	Oxygen consumption at max effort	Sustained oxygen utilization
Intensity	High intensity	Moderate intensity
Fuel source	Glycogen primarily	Fat and glycogen mix
Adaptations	Cardiovascular, respiratory	Metabolic, muscular
Training type	HIIT, intervals	Steady-state, LSD

Aerobic cardio

- **Definition: Aerobic cardio refers to exercise sustained over a long period at moderate intensity, relying primarily on oxygen for energy production. This zone is where fat is burned.**

Scientific basis

- **Utilizes fat and carbohydrates as fuel through oxidative metabolism.**
- Efficiency depends on mitochondrial density, capillary supply, and enzymatic activity in muscles.

Real-world example

- **Long-distance running, cycling, or swimming at a pace where conversation is still possible.**

- Example: Running a 10K at 60–75% of maximum heart rate.

Training aerobic cardio

- **Steady-state training**
  - Prolonged exercise at a consistent pace.
  - Examples: A 90-minute zone 2 run or a 2-hour bike ride at moderate effort.

- **LSD (Long Slow Distance)**
  - Running or cycling at low intensity for extended periods.
  - Builds endurance by enhancing fat metabolism and increasing mitochondrial efficiency.

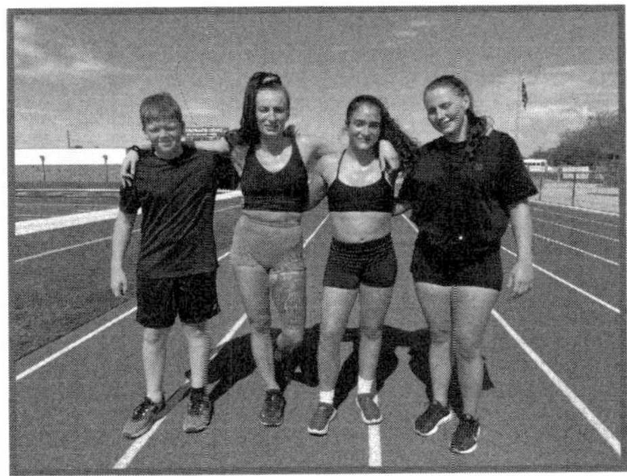

On Saturdays we sprint. Even my son comes out. And there's no better plyo in the world than fast sprints—especially 400m's!

Seigher Brown

VO_2 max (maximal oxygen uptake)

- **Definition: VO_2 Max is the maximum rate at which your body can uptake, transport, and utilize oxygen during intense exercise. It is a key indicator of cardiorespiratory fitness.**

- **VO_2:** Volume of oxygen consumed.
- **Max:** Maximum limit during exercise.

Scientific basis

- **Expressed as milliliters of oxygen consumed per kilogram of body weight per minute (ml/kg/min).**
- Reflects the efficiency of the heart, lungs, and muscles in oxygen utilization.

Real-world example

- **Elite endurance athletes like marathoners or cyclists often have VO_2 Max values above 70 ml/kg/min.**
- A sedentary individual may have a VO_2 Max around 30–40 ml/kg/min.

Training VO_2 max

- **High-intensity interval training (HIIT) is one of the most effective methods.**
- Example: Perform 4–6 reps of 3–5 min at 90–95% of maximal heart rate, with equal rest periods.

- Gradual overload and progression are essential to push physiological limits.
- Activities: Sprint intervals, cycling, rowing, swimming, hill running.

MORE THAN RUNNING

All the examples above, whether zone 2 or VO_2 max training, are all incorporated through running exercises, but there's zero need to run at all—though I do think running is very important.

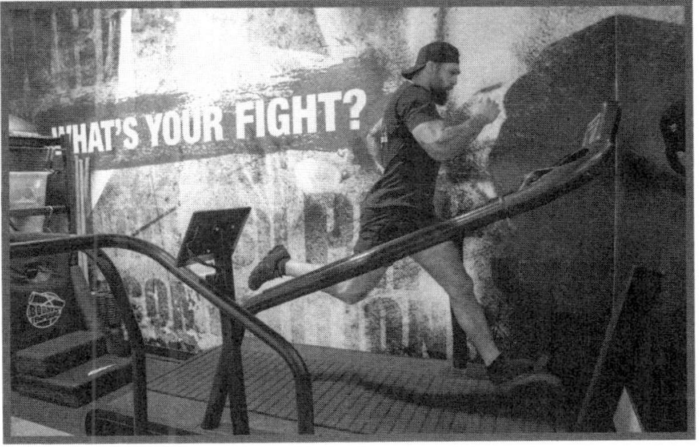

Sprinting with intent of form—driving forward versus up and down will significantly improve running speed. *Seigher Brown*

In MMA, your zone 2 training could be skills work. Bret Contreras says, "Why just run? There's only so much time in the day, and you could hit the bag, shadowbox, work ground and pound—or any other skills work for your zone 2." The key, though, is wearing a heart rate monitor and adhering to your maximal heart rate to stay within the zone 2 parameter. It's very easy to get excited while punching or kicking (or even shadowboxing!) and all of a sudden, your heart rate shoots up to 165 bpm and you're no longer expanding your aerobic base.

For Kamuela's last UFC fight, we implemented various 45- to 60-min training sessions and mixed it up between slow runs, slow bike rides, and bag work (both standing and ground and pound). He lost his last UFC fight, but said, "I know I lost, but it was the best I've ever physically felt in any of my fights. I know I was tired, but I would have never been able to push like that in the third round like I did in this fight."

The same concept for zone 2 can be implemented for VO_2 max efforts as well. Maximal effort doesn't have to be a run. Sprinting is a great way to push your heart rate to failure, and it's a great way to control the situation, as trying to spike your heart rate with weights or live sports training can be a quick way to an injury, but there are a ton of other ways to push the VO_2 boundary.

Ballistic circuits (sandbag lifts and throws, frog/broad jumps), aerodyne sprints, versa climbers, and 400-m sprints are all great VO_2 max exercises which can be performed with a relatively low risk of injury. The key to VO_2 max efforts, just like plyometrics, is max effort. If athletes aren't resting enough in between rounds or sets, they aren't pushing into their max effort and are in a sub–zone 5 max effort phase. If you're wanting to run fast, but are too tired, you're just jogging—which is fine when we want to jog, but not when we want to sprint.

One of my favorite training sessions I've seen transfer almost immediately to the mats and cage is 400-m sprints. Go to the track and get a few laps as a warm-up. Then run through some movement prep: A-skips, B-skips etc. And then sprint 400 m. The first time you run these, you're going to completely overdo the first 200–300 m and you're going to hit a wall before you even finish the first lap. Running 400 m is a different pace than running 100 m or 200 m. But you'll figure it out. So, run the 400 m. I then let my fighters REST AS LONG AS THEY NEED TO IN ORDER TO RUN ANOTHER SPRINT WITH THE SAME INTENSITY. Repeat. Rarely can anyone get more than three working laps on the first track session. Four is unbelievably impressive. I've never seen five on a first attempt. There is nothing like the max effort of a 400-m sprint. Your lungs are on fire. Your legs and shoulders are scorched. Everything hurts, but you push through. Then you collapse when you hit the finish line.

During Henry Cejudo's second training camp for a title shot against

Demetrious Johnson, we knew we had to go to extreme efforts. We had to be able to push for 25 minutes against one of the best to have ever stepped in a cage. Demetrious never got tired. He was extremely fast. And he was good. Like really, really . . . really good! In my opinion, he's the most technical fighter to have ever fought. It was my favorite fight to game-plan for—there was a riddle in front of me, and I had to match Henry's strengths and weaknesses vs Demetrious's strengths and weaknesses. Separate from the tactical approaches we needed to decipher, we also had a physical component to overcome—we needed Henry to be able to fight—hard.

Our gym owner, Dave Zowine, brought on board a team of trainers from a company called NeuroForce 1. They brought science to another level. None of us had seen this type of attention to detail before. Every workout was monitored via heart rate. Every morning, Henry's recovery was measured by a machine called the Omegawave—a contraption with electrodes that attached to his chest, arms, and even head. It was like an EKG met an EEG, and it measured Heart Rate Variability, stress levels, blood pressure, and a slew of other physical attributes.

NeuroForce brought so much science to the table, but what stood out most were the short, max effort bursts of VO_2 pushes. I mentioned above that pushing for VO_2 max efforts via sports training is dangerous, as there's an increased risk of injury, but we went for it. For these pushes, Henry was scheduled for 20 max effort goes. He was tasked with sparring or wrestling (he's such a good wrestler, and one of the few people whose heart rate generally lowers during wrestling), depending on the day and goal, for one-minute pushes once his HR rose to over 185 bpm. Sometimes his HR would reach higher, but he had to maintain that workload for a minute. Then he'd rest until his heart rate hit 148 bpm—a 20% decrease. It could take him an hour or ten seconds to hit that number, and then we'd go again. The 20% decrease was based on how recovered we hoped he'd become during the minute rest between each round of the fight. After weeks of this type of training, Henry was able to maintain extended periods with very high heart rates (180–190 bpm), but he was also recovering 22–25% during the 1-minute breaks in between sparring rounds.

Separately, for reference, we also didn't adhere to the "1-minute rest" between sparring rounds during his camp, but rather used a heart rate monitor and always started the next round as soon as his heart rate had recovered to that 20% number (20% of his max HR during the previous round). We wanted his body to adapt faster, and by using the 20% recovery method, we always knew exactly when he was as recovered as we needed him to be. Fortunately, Henry won that Demetrious fight by split decision. His cardio looked amazing, and he was now the UFC Flyweight world champion.

COMBINING VO_2 MAX AND AEROBIC TRAINING

I truly believe VO_2 max and zone 2 work should be trained separately. Our bodies are so much more efficient than our knowledge base of sports science, but if you are going to combine them in a form of HIIT training, I prefer a modified version. A very common form of HIIT treadmill work would consist of a warm-up run and then a base run. Warm up for five minutes, and then increase the speed to, say, 7 mph for three minutes. After those three minutes, increase the speed to 9 mph for a minute. Once the minute is finished, drop the speed to 7.2 mph. Then it increases to 9.2 mph, and drops to 7.4 mph for three minutes. It will then go to 9.2 mph for a minute, and then drop to 7.6 mph, and so on and so forth. This increases the output for the base run and the sprint.

I prefer a different approach. I like to find a speed on the treadmill that my fighter can maintain at approximately 145–150 bpm. Jog at that speed for 3 minutes to start, and then push the speed and incline as high as possible—where my fighter can maintain the effort for 30 seconds. Then decrease the speed. Allow the fighter's heart rate to recover to the 145–150 bpm and maintain that for 3 minutes and then sprint again. If the fighter can continue after the 30 seconds, the speed or incline should be increased. Both have their respective advantages: In my observation, increasing the incline tends to push the muscles harder, whereas increasing the speed tends to tax the lungs more. Repeat this process ten times.

Yet another VO_2 max training style is that of the Swedes, where they will run 80–90% max for 3–4 minute pushes—really tax their system—and then walk for an equal time to their work time. They repeat this 3–5 times. So, if you run as hard (almost as hard, so you can maintain) as you can for 4 minutes, you then walk for 4 minutes. Repeat that four times. The total time will be approximately 32 minutes, and these are aimed at increasing your VO_2 max.

Note on sprinting: quick note on the importance of sprinting and zone 2

Most S&C coaches will not program sprinting into an MMA athlete's routine. I highly disagree with this.

Like I mentioned earlier, sprinting is the ultimate plyometric exercise. If you are truly fast (running a sub–5-second 40-yard dash) you are going to jump high and be dynamic.

Second, the faster you can sprint, the less energy you're expending relative to your slower opponents. If you and your opponent's max speed on a sprint is 10 mph, and you're running at 80% your max, well that's 8 mph and your heart rate will be higher at 80% max speed than, say, 70% max speed.

If you can run 20 mph max speed, and you're running at 8 mph with your opponent, well, you're only running at 40% your max speed, and your heart rate will be much slower.

It's all about effort in relation to your maximal abilities. Be faster, and then you work less any time you're not at max speed in relation to being slower.

Last, many S&C coaches want to keep weight training programmed late into fight camps. "Ballistic/power/speed tends to deteriorate after two weeks" blah, blah, blah. Yes, that is all true, but true power and strength and whatnot is not what a fighter cares about or needs late in fight camp, it's cardio—whether muscular endurance or VO_2 max or recoverability, it's cardio. But sprinting is a way to cheat all of this a bit. If an athlete is really working sprint work into a routine, she's getting some of that dynamic work that will be removed from other exercises. Just make sure there's a buildup, as trying to max sprint without building a base and building up to the workload is a surefire way to pull a hamstring!

Zone 2

The more time we spend in zone 2 during practice, the greater our aerobic base, which makes our time in zones 3/4/5 more efficient and allows for faster recovery in those zones.

Remember: zone 2 is making our cells work more efficiently. How? Well, when our body is in zone 2, it increases the size and the efficiency of the mitochondria, which is the part of the cell where glycogen is broken down into ATP—the energy source we use in our higher heart ranges.

By having a larger zone 2 base, it doesn't mean we are going to necessarily stay in lower zones during high-intensity training. What it means is that our bodies will be more efficient with their energy systems while in those zones. And, of course, we can recover faster after those high zones are hit because of our aerobic capacity to transfer oxygen back to our muscles. Zone 2 is the recovery for the work done at VO_2 max or higher zones.

And remember, it's not always the fastest person who wins the race, but the one who slows down last.

10

THE HOLISTIC APPROACH

Definition
Holistic—ho·lis·tic
/hōˈlistik/
adjective

"characterized by the belief that the parts of something are interconnected and can be explained only by reference to the whole."[1]

Being exceptional somewhere means being deficient somewhere else. Show me the richest man in the world, and I'll show you someone who sacrificed in other aspects to achieve that success.

If the last two chapters were about defining different types of exercise, this chapter explains how they work with one another. To use a clichéd but understandable analogy, if you have the absolute best road bike in the world, but you have a flat tire, the rest of the bike can't operate to its full ability. If the gear system goes out, the fastest tires and suspension system don't matter. If the chain breaks, you have a beautiful paperweight. All those components are, seemingly, very separate from one another, but each is key for overall performance. The human body is exactly the same. Strength without speed, power without cardio, speed without recoverability will lead to performance deficiencies. In addition to a holistic approach to the body, you also need a holistic approach to training—which means your coaches need to fit the right piece of the pie as well. All too often, every single coach wants every single bit of energy out of their athlete at every practice, which causes overlap and major training gaps as well. If your strength coach kills your legs in the weight room, how are you supposed to do a full speed PR on the track that afternoon with your running coach? Communication is key. Balance is key. Understanding goals, both short- and long-term, is key.

As Dr. Roman Fomin, the Senior Director of Performance Science at the UFC Performance Institute, explains, "I also recommend that they take a holistic approach because we are working with one athlete with one biological system and that system is taking multiple different training sessions and working with multiple specialists, so it's very important to understand the overall training load that we put on that fighter . . . Our fighters are very dedicated, but I would say a more structured approach and better connection between technical and nontechnical training sessions will further their development."

When UFC fighter Kamuela Kirk was having major cardio/conditioning issues when his fights ran into the later rounds, we had to make adjustments, as there was an imbalance in his physiology. His natural power and explosiveness were an asset early in fights but became a detriment as the fight progressed—he didn't have the aerobic capacity or ability to buffer lactic acid needed to perform late in the fight. First, we disassembled Kamuela's strength routine, which other coaches prescribed: "more lactate pushes," "more reps," "harder pushes," and "fight-simulating circuits." Then we switched instead to a pure strength program focusing on specific muscle groups with large, compound movements. He lifted, rested for a period of time, and then performed another set. Rinse and repeat. We went back in time to the 1990s at any local Gold's gym and took how the gym bros were lifting back then. Sometimes new isn't better! Then we added zone 2 cardio, which was having him run so slow he had to almost speed walk—the complete opposite of what the strength and conditioning specialists were prescribing. But it worked.

Increasing Kamuela's overall strength allowed him to tap into the slower moving (less energy expenditure) muscles used in a lot of his grappling. He didn't rely on those big explosive movements to get himself out of trouble. And because he was physically stronger, he didn't get into *as much* trouble from opponents being able to move him around and compromise his position, and he could move others around. His heart rate didn't spike as high during grappling exchanges, either, but when it did, his aerobic capacity was greater, which allowed for faster recovery and lactic buffering to occur, so he wasn't in need of rest. He didn't need to take time off before attacking again or exchanging in scrambles.

These examples are just a glimpse of how the holistic approach is paramount in athletic performance. Athletes need the proper strength and conditioning for their body. They need the proper skills training for their sport. They need the proper periodization for their training camp, which will often start with filling the gaps of deficiencies and then moving into different phases (strength, power, speed, lactic thresholds), and maybe back and forth a few times before the competition date. We don't live in a vacuum in any aspect of our lives. We shouldn't live in one in our athletic endeavors either.

IF WE'RE TOO CLOSE TO THE TREE, WE CAN'T SEE THE FOREST.

This whole book is an example of the holistic approach. You can take each chapter as a stand-alone, and tremendously educate yourself on a topic of choice. However, you'd be doing yourself a disservice to do just that. When we discuss recovery, we must discuss our load management of strength and conditioning. If we increase our weights too quickly, we're likely to become injured and overtrained. Managing the progressive overload of our strength helps us manage our recovery. Trying to manage our recovery but ignoring our overloaded work rate is just like trying to save money by cutting out our Starbucks when our mortgage is $8,000/mo. Trying to work cardio and improve your VO_2 max without proper nutrition is almost comical—especially if you're on a low-carb diet and don't have the energy to walk up a set of stairs, let alone push your heart rate to its absolute max.

Everything works together in a synchronized, harmonious fashion with our body. Our brains signal to the endocrine system to release hormones, and then our circulatory system (blood) carries those hormones to our digestive system or skin or muscles (all different systems). If any one of those systems fails, the others can't perform their duty. And there's a good chance we die . . . but that's a different book.

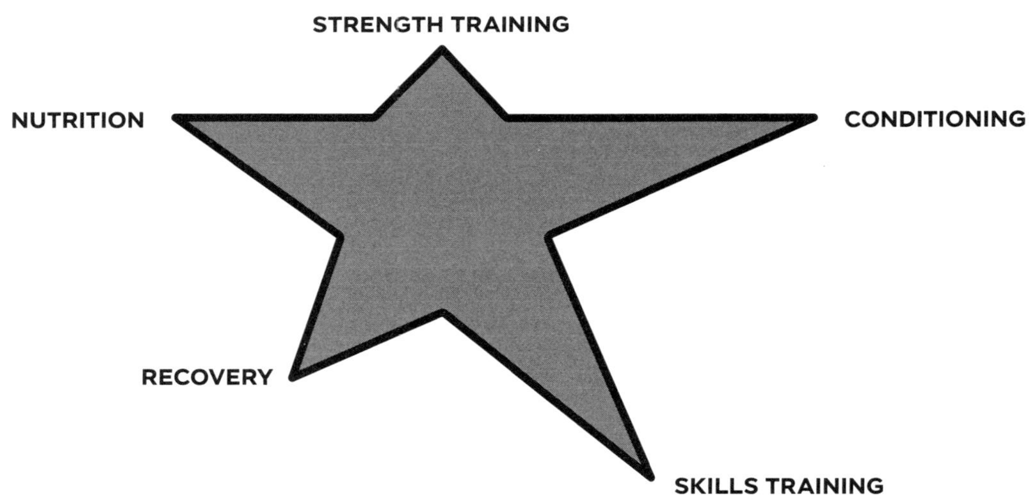

THE WEAKEST LINK

A chain is only as strong as its weakest link, and an athlete is only as strong as his weakest deficiency. You will absolutely win some fights and games and races at the lower level or even at a moderate level by having that one superhuman trait. I see it all the time with my sons' youth wrestling. A kid can be down by ten points, but he finds that one move he's good at and wins by cradle. Another kid is talented on a technical level, but the other kids have started puberty and are so much more physical, and the talented kid doesn't have a shot. But eventually, our deficiencies catch up to us. Look at Paulo Costa in the UFC. He was a KO machine, but once people figured out that his cardio fades in the later rounds, they knew how to beat him. One of my fighters, Jonathan Pearce, who I mentioned earlier, came into the UFC and put together five wins in a row after his debut loss, but had some holes in his submission grappling game, and has lost three fights since. We push him constantly to get into Brazilian Jiu Jitsu classes, but we haven't been successful, and now we're staring down the wrong end of a UFC record and trajectory.

Much of the gains we make, as athletes, are more about fixing deficiencies than adding gains, but we don't always see the deficiencies at face value. Like Kamuela: His lactate threshold was failing him at his VO_2 max level, but it wasn't because of the VO_2 max; rather, it was because he didn't have the zone 2 to support that max. Athletic deficiencies often present themselves as more of a riddle than a science. It's as if we're all watching a *House, M.D.* episode trying to figure

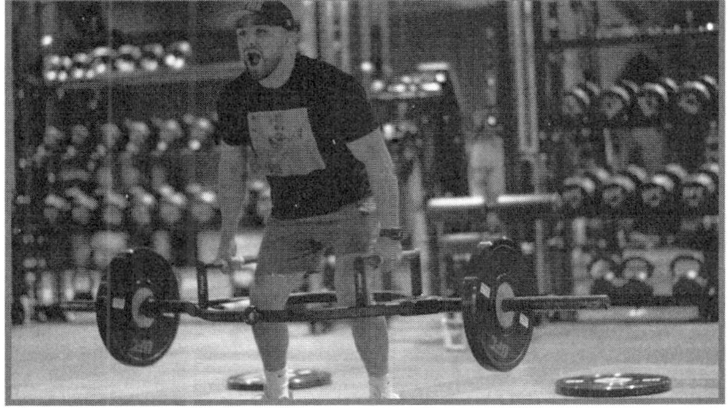

Weak links break chains. Using compound movements is a great way to reduce deficiencies in areas. *Seigher Brown*

out why the woman on the hospital bed is dying, when none of it makes sense. And just like on *House, M.D.*, the answer is often simple, but we're just looking in the wrong place.

HOLISTIC ATHLETIC OPTIMIZATION FRAMEWORK

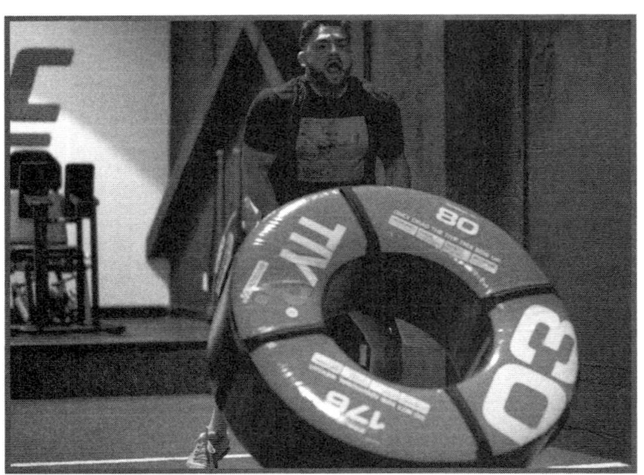

Tire flips are the "next best thing" to cleans. They are a safer way for newer lifters to throw really heavy things in the air with their entire body. *Seigher Brown*

Dr. Roman Fomin calls everything I'm telling you the Holistic Athletic Optimization Framework, and although it's a mouthful, it's very useful to hear him break down exactly how each piece of the puzzle fits together—when your puzzle is an athlete, and the puzzle pieces are made up of every detail for that athlete to compete at her highest level.

Dr. Fomin emphasizes a systems-based approach that integrates **physical readiness**, **mental resilience**, and **data-driven adaptability**. His philosophy rejects one-dimensional training in favor of synchronized development across seven physiological systems (cardiac, respiratory, metabolic, muscular, skeletal, nervous, and brain function). He breaks these down into three main pillars:

1. **Physiological system syncing**
    - Athletes must balance stress/recovery cycles across interdependent systems.

- Example: Heavy dead lifts stress nervous/muscular systems—follow with low-intensity, low stress work the following day.
- *"You can't overstimulate the same systems daily. If Monday fries your nervous system, Tuesday should focus on recovered systems like cardio."*

2. **Tiered diagnostic testing**

   UFC PI uses 3-tier assessments:

- **Tier 1:** Body comp, resting metabolism, orthopedic screening.
- **Tier 2:** Sport-specific tests (10×6 sled pushes with gas/breath analysis, loaded CMJ (countermovement) jumps, neck assessments).
- **Tier 3:** Longitudinal tracking of HRV trends and fight-specific biomarkers.
- *"We identify 'flat tires'—if you're 15% below weight class averages in anaerobic sustainability, that becomes camp priority #1."*

3. **Brain-centric performance**

   Fomin considers the nervous system the ultimate bottleneck:

- It trains "neural reserves" through mindfulness protocols.
- It uses Omegawave-style EEG/ECG combos to track brain-heart coherence.
- *"The brain can suppress or facilitate performance. We've barely scratched unlocking its fight IQ potential."*

These are the UFC's testing protocols, but you may have a very different protocol for your sport or goal. Are you a receiver with great top end speed, but you don't accelerate well? Do you fatigue in the second half? As a defensive end, you may want your max sled push for 50 yards to increase. The real takeaway here is finding your deficiency and working toward improving it. By filling the hole left by that deficiency, you let other systems operate at full capacity, and you can work on excelling, as opposed to not failing (somewhere else).

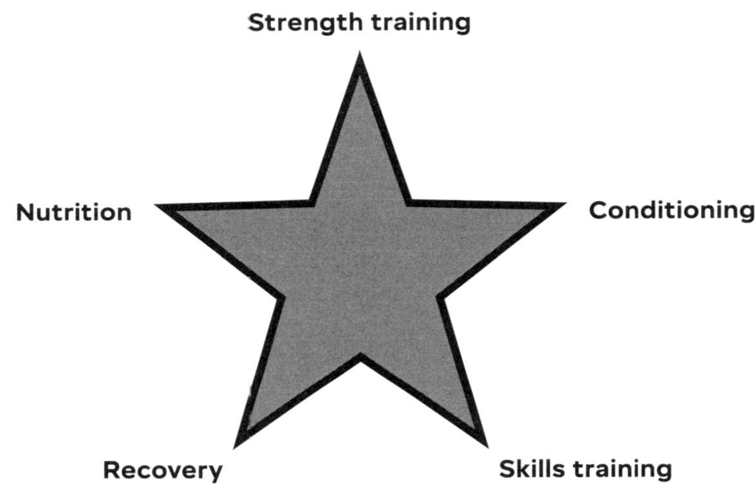

PRACTICAL APPLICATIONS

I don't want to just give theory. I want you to leave here with some sort of understanding on how to go about fixing some common deficiencies that might occur during your athletic endeavors. This is by no means exhaustive. By the very nature of this book, I'm going against my own principles because each and every one of you is going to have a different physiology; therefore, the answer to these problems is going to be different. Take myself for example and compare me to Kamuela because you have already heard a lot about him. Earlier in my career I would become tired in the third round, just like Kamuela, but where his was more his zone 2 aerobic base couldn't keep up with the power and dynamic movements he put his body through, mine was because I didn't have the muscular strength base (and to a lesser degree, technical wrestling base) to push hard in those final five minutes, but I had all the zone 2 cardio anyone could ask for.

We both had the same "problem" of fatigue in the third round, but the cause was completely different for us, and if we tried to solve the problem with the same answer, one of us would surely not benefit. So take the following with a very small grain of salt, and use them as general ideas because I don't know you, and I don't know what problems you're having with your athletic career.

Below are some tips to help in the most common deficit areas. These aren't workouts, per se, but you can easily build a workout around these helpful knowledge points!

DEFICITS

Muscular endurance

Examples: rower, skier, mountain climber, horse jockey, wrestler, MMA fighter

If you find your arms and legs are shaking and weak when you try to climb or ride a horse and they are giving out, you need to improve your muscular endurance, but I wouldn't start there. Reverse-engineer the situation, and first, ensure you are strong enough in your fundamental Olympic lifts (bench, squat, dead lift) and capable of performing 10–15 pull-ups. You're going to want an overall higher strength base, which will make it easier to apply the endurance phase. Spend the first four weeks working Olympic strength lifts and reach for the higher end of the rep range for strength of 6 reps, and even teeter into the 6–8 rep range.

Then move into a muscular endurance phase, consisting of 20–25 reps per set. My rule of thumb for this phase is if you can't get to 20 reps, the weight is too heavy. If you can get to 26 reps, the weight is too light. Start with a full-body workout—one exercise per muscle group (quad, hamstring, glute, upper body push, upper body pull). If you've ever performed a set of dead lifts or squats to failure in the 20–25 rep range (like actual failure—legs shaking about to fall over failure), you know how exhausting this will be. Your body will be fried. Perform one set per body part, three days a week. After the first week, if you feel you can increase to two sets per body part, do so. Work your way up to three sets per body part, and then get back on that horse or ski or whatever, and your muscles will not be failing you!

Bonus: Isometric holds. In the athletic world, everyone tends to cater toward the dynamic, the power, the speed—which is great for soccer and football, but isometric, static holds are amazing at building muscular endurance. And not all sports are dynamic based! Weighted wall sits, dumbbell farmer's carries, chin up/pull-up holds for 30 seconds (or longer) are great ways to create muscular endurance.

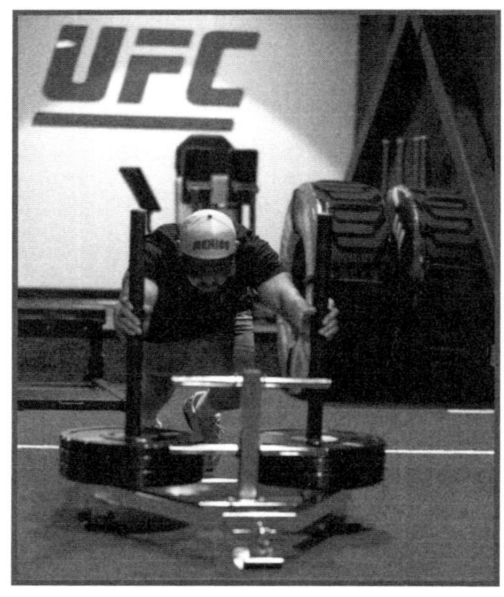

Farmer walks and sled pushes are both great for getting you strong—moving heavy weight for extended periods of time stresses the muscles and nervous system.

Seigher Brown

Strength

Examples: lineman, wrestler, basketball player (being pushed around and not being able to stand your ground)

One of the biggest issues I see with people who try to get stronger is they try to skip steps and go too fast. They want that number on the bar, but they're not ready for it. They don't create the foundation to push that weight. Just as with muscular endurance needing a strength base, strength needs a muscular endurance base—"same same, but different," as my Mongolian fighters say to us.

To get stronger, you don't want to raise the reps to the muscular endurance range of 20–25, but you will want to start with 8–10 reps, which is generally more reps than strength-focused athletes and coaches would prescribe, and teeters into the hypertrophy (bodybuilding/mass gain) range of lifting weights. But if you want to get stronger, a better base is needed first, and extra size most likely won't hurt. Just be careful with your overall load, as the higher reps will most likely lead to more DOMS, and depending on whether you're in season/camp or out of season/camp, this may be detrimental for performance. Remember, the minimum effective dose is key to avoiding DOMS.

When faced with a problem, too many people attack it head-on, and that isn't always the answer. Remember, many people have an underlying deficiency that needs to be brought up—strengthening the overall base before a specific area of focus can be improved. When faced with a strength deficit, too many people start with reps of 3–4 trying to get their one-rep-max number higher too quickly.

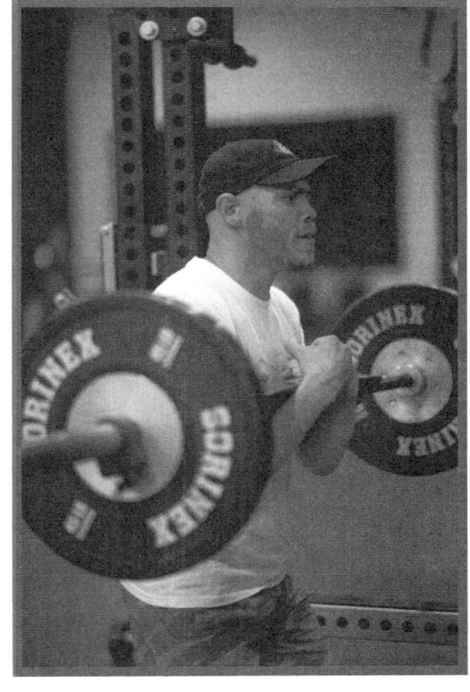

Zercher squats are a great mix between a deadlift and squat and work both the hamstring and quad as opposed to a traditional squat that limits hamstring activation. *Seigher Brown*

If you are in season, absolutely perform full-body workouts, as opposed to trying to hit upper/lower body split. This will help keep overall time in the weight room down, and will help limit reps/sets, i.e. DOMS. If you're not in season, go full send and be as sore as you want, as long as you're not so sore it keeps you out of the gym. Soreness is a horrible indicator of both the load side and the recovery side. Being sore is just . . . well, being sore.

With overall strength being your goal, try to

perform lower/upper compound movements first, and more often. Cleans, dead lifts, sled push/pulls, and farmer walks inside the trap bar are going to render the greatest ROI. Always begin with the movements that have the greater risk of injury, dead lifts, and finish each session with farmer walks, which are such a full-body scorcher!

Don't forget about isolation lifts here. If time isn't an issue—especially out of season/camp—isolation lifts can have amazing results on your compound numbers. Strength coach Matt Wiedemer regularly loves to overload the triceps if people are having a difficult time with their bench press numbers. Oftentimes it's not the pectoral muscles not being able to push the load, but rather the triceps muscles are the weak link. The same might go for squat and deadlift numbers. Maybe it's the forearm muscles and grip strength causing the breakdown in the dead lift, or the glutes are too weak for the squat or even vice versa. Remember, everything works together!

CARDIO: TIRED DOWN THE STRETCH

Cardio is tricky. This is the one that gets everyone in trouble because what are we actually talking about when we say "cardio"? Do we mean our aerobic cardio? VO_2 max? Muscular endurance? All we know is we felt tired and couldn't push any farther. We're limited by our own understanding of what "cardio" we're even talking about, let alone our ability to articulate it in coherent terms for another human to understand. We're toddlers yelling, "My tummy hurts!" And mommy is trying to figure out if that means we have gas or have the flu or if we were punched or if something is internally wrong with us—all we know is our tummy hurts and we want mommy to fix it—not knowing she is completely unable to help as, one, she can't even decipher what our problem is, and two, even if she could get to the root cause, she's fiercely unqualified to do anything about it. And that's our strength and conditioning conundrum with cardio and athletes fatiguing during competition. Athletes can't describe what's failing them, and coaches can't do anything about it anyway. So here we are.

As mentioned, cardio, for the most part, consists of your zone 2 and your VO_2 max. Everything else in between is of no consequence to me here. Yes, all are important, but these two zones are the ones I care about.

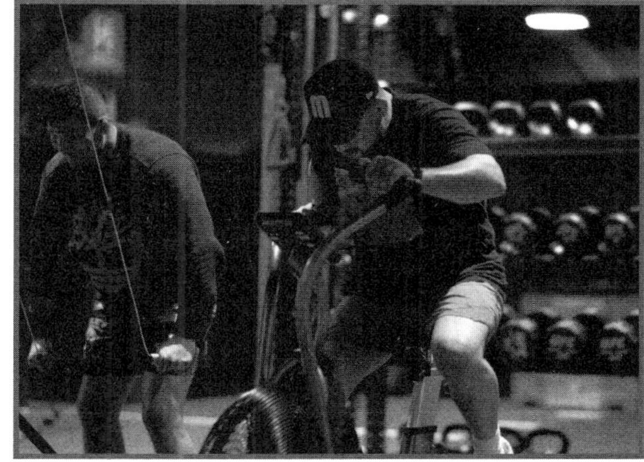

Assault/fan bikes spike the heart rate and tax every muscle in your body. Nobody enjoys them. *Seigher Brown*

If we've already ruled out muscular endurance and strength training as a possible fix, then we are, indeed, talking cardio. You need to work with both zone 2 and VO_2 max in tandem to figure out what the real problem is, and chances are, it's probably some sort of combination of the two. Remember, zone 2 is your base, so your VO_2 max can only get as tall as the pyramid's base will allow.

Are you an athlete who's getting tired on the fourth lap in a mile run down the stretch or an athlete getting tired in the third period of a wrestling match? I can't, definitively, tell anyone what they need in either scenario without meeting with them and running tests, but I'd hazard a guess: Do the opposite of what you currently spend most of your time doing on a regular basis.

A wrestler is going to hit the VO_2 max range just about every single day in practice. She's going to push her body for 10, 20, 45 seconds at a time and maintain a frenetic pace all the while. She isn't lacking those max effort bursts. But if she's getting tired during matches, maybe she should work on her zone

2 cardio. Long, light runs (bike rides or elliptical are fine too, though I always believe running is better) where she can hold a conversation are best. Forty-five minutes to an hour, three to five days a week. She won't be sore, and her training should be only moderately altered to handle the additional workload.

However, if our runner is used to putting the miles in, if he's used to running 3, 5, even 10 miles at a time, maybe he needs the opposite prescription. How often is he pushing himself to max effort failure? He should implement some 400-m sprints into his regimen as well as some 200-m and even 100-m sprints. He might need to push himself to complete failure. He already has the aerobic base, now he needs to push his heart rate to the max.

ONE LAST THING

When all else fails, don't forget about the main thing. If you want to run faster, sprint. If you want to jump higher, jump. If you want to punch harder, punch things. If you want to get stronger, lift things.

11

RECOVERY

THE QUICK VERSION FIRST

The topic of recovery has become a thorn in my side over the last few years because it's almost not real. We're talking fake news here. Unicorns and leprechauns. Mountains out of molehills.

- **Are you working too hard? Did you add too much training load and intensity too quickly to your program? Did you allow enough rest between intense days of training?**

- Are you sleeping well? Do you go to bed at the same time and wake up at the same time every day, or do you stay up all night playing video games and scrolling social media?

- Are you eating well? Are your meals balanced with proteins, complex carbs, vegetables, and some fats?

- Are you stressed? If you're focusing on too many variables out of your control, you're going to create anxiety and you won't recover.

THAT'S PRETTY MUCH IT, FOLKS. WE'RE DONE HERE!

Those four bullet points are pretty much the 90% rule of recovery, but we like to overcomplicate things. We really don't need to go on, but we will.

First let's talk about the difference between athletic performance recovery and athletic function recovery.

Athletic performance recovery is what I describe as *how* we're competing from one day to the next. How recovered an athlete is from yesterday to today after performing a level of physical activity, and what level her physical and mental readiness to train is at following the period of rest and recovery. That could be comparing our sprint speeds or times, how high we could jump last week to this week, how much we lifted then vs now, or how well we sparred yesterday compared with how well we spar tomorrow. Generally, these are quantifiable attributes we can measure; however, in combat sports the intended outcomes for success aren't necessarily quantifiable, so we need to use a more qualitative analysis of our performance (not how we feel).

Athletic function recovery is more of a qualitative analysis of how we're *feeling*. Am I sore? Can my joints move in a full range of motion? Am I flexible? Is there a knot in my muscle? Do I feel like training?

As a coach, I don't really care about athletic function recovery. I absolutely understand how important feeling good means to athletic success, but "feeling good" isn't quantifiable, and just as the decrease in DOMS isn't a valid indicator of being recovered and being exhausted/sore isn't a valid indicator of a workout being productive, feeling good or bad rarely translates into athletic performance one way or the other. What I do care about is HRV (if we're tracking it) and max heart rate—a very early sign of overtraining is if an athlete's heart rate won't get above 160–165 bpm. I care about athletic function recovery and I also care about numerous other factors during camp when training load and recovery need to be considered, but "feeling good," "being sore," "having muscle tightness or knots" are for a massage therapist or a life partner to handle. I'm here to handle training, whether we "feel" good or not.

Now, let's not get confused. Whether we're measuring our HRV via wearable monitor or not, I absolutely want to hear if someone feels READY to train. You know your body. If you feel physically taxed or mentally taxed or a cold/flu coming on, that is a "feeling" I care about. Feeling "ready and able" is very different than feeling "sore or lethargic." Subtle differences in language, huge differences of intent.

Christmas morning

Recovery is simple, but simple isn't always monetizable, and people want your money; they want my money. They want to commercialize every holiday so our spending goes up and up and up. Love and affection don't create profits. Less doesn't create profits. Just more. Recovery in sports is like buying your children toys for their birthday and for Christmas. They open gift after gift after gift—so many toys, we must love our kids so much—look how many we bought them! We go into their rooms a week or month later and there are toys on the shelves. Toys in the closet. Toys under the bed. A mess of toys everywhere. But the toys are all there because little Suzy only plays with the one Barbie and a toy lawnmower. The rest are just there. Unused, but they keep the room full. If mommy tried to throw them away, Suzy would throw a fit. They look good. The logic seems that she'd want more toys. The more she has, the more games she can play. The more mommy and daddy feel validated, just like your S&C coach seeks validation. Just like the companies you're buying from seek your dollars. But more than anything, you feel validated if you have an answer for what "more" you can do to recover. We want answers, even if the answer is wrong—having a positive sum (an answer) is easier for humans than having a negative sum ("I don't know the answer" or "do nothing," i.e., no answer). Filling that void of where the answer should go seems like it should be "something" as opposed to "nothing."

We need to stop demanding answers for everything that may not have a positive sum answer. We ask our coach, "How do I recover?" Coach says, "Rest." We don't like that answer, so we leave coach and find a new coach. Now, the next time our old coach is asked the same question, he's going to give a different answer. He'll suggest something because if he doesn't, he'll go out of business.

WHAT'S NOT RECOVERY

So before we dive deeper into recovery, here are some things that aren't recovery:

1. Ice baths/cryotherapy: Ice baths have numerous benefits such as stress reduction and inflammation reduction, but you don't need an ice bath for recovery, and actually, if you take an ice bath within a few hours of any sort of hypertrophy training, you may as well have never lifted in the first place. Ice reduces inflammation, but the inflammatory process is paramount in the breaking down and rebuilding of muscle tissue fiber.

   Ice is, however, great for acute recovery—you're running a relay race and need to reduce inflammation before your next leg of the race is up.

   As for athletic performance, you're not going to be getting much here.

2. Massage guns: Nope. There's pretty much zero support that massage guns aid in recovery whatsoever. They do feel great! But they aren't really helping you recover. To a somewhat lesser extent, that foam roller isn't helping either, but there are studies that show DOMS is reduced by using a foam roller, and range of motion might be improved with the use of foam rollers shortly after workouts. Athletic performance, though? Nope.

3. Compression boots: Normatec boots and similar products are supposed to squeeze lactic acid out of the muscles and aid in recovery. They feel great. I use them regularly as my legs regularly feel achy and stiff, but they aren't going to help me recover either.

4. Massage: Massages are great for athletes. They are great to break up myofascial buildup and to keep athletes feeling loose and limber, but they aren't going to speed up an athlete's ability to sprint at max effort any sooner than he would with rest.

LOOK AT RECOVERY AS A STEROID

A simplistic approach to the "is it recovery or not" debate is to look at recovery through the lens of a steroid, or even a hormone like testosterone or HGH because, at the most profound level, that's how steroids work: They speed up recovery. Steroid abusers in sports have the advantage because they can train more than the natural athlete. The steroid abuser can work out to max effort, go to sleep, and be almost fully recovered the next day, whereas the natural athlete needs a few days to recover before he's able to train at the same intensity again. Steroids grow muscle back faster, so you can lift more, sooner. You can sprint 3× a week instead of 2×. That's the advantage.

If we look at recovery as a steroid, will a massage gun grow my muscles back any faster? Will an ice bath replenish my glycogen levels in my muscles? Will a red light or PEMF (Pulsed Electromagnetic Field) mat add more red blood cells to my body?

Now, if I do nothing but rest, will my body repair itself? If I sleep well, will my body produce more testosterone and HGH, compounds we know expedite recovery and muscle/tissue growth? If I eat adequate amounts of proteins and carbohydrates, will my body break those compounds down and use them to fuel my cells and regenerate my broken-down tissues?

LET'S DIVE DEEPER, THOUGH

Sleep, workload management, and a balanced diet are the real performance enhancing drugs (i.e., recovery)!

Gains are made during recovery.

If you've trained for any reasonable amount of time, you've probably heard this saying, and although a bit overused, it is very true. The body has a natural cycle to deal with exercise and recovery just as it does for every process. While awake, our brains build up waste and toxins, and when we sleep those toxins are flushed out. When we eat, we start with chewing, then digesting, then absorption, and then excretion. During exercise, we perform an athletic task, then our bodies must repair themselves and discard the waste created during that process. We must take out the trash in our house or it builds up into a dump. The same is true with our bodies.

Let me start with three examples. First, the standard, basic version that you've probably heard: Lifting weights results in muscle fibers breaking down. The body immediately begins to repair those torn fibers over the current muscle, resulting in a bigger, stronger muscle than before. If, instead of resting that muscle, it works again the next day, the muscle never has time to fully repair, and it's broken down again and again until it has time to recover. This is why recovery is key—the gains are developed during recovery.

The second example is during training. I often have my fighters run 400-m sprints. The fighters warm up with a few laps around the track and then begin to sprint in 400-m increments. If they do well, most will clock the lap around 1–1:15 minutes. Ideally, each subsequent lap shouldn't drop too much in time/speed, and I give a long time in between laps—pretty much as much time as needed before the fighters run another lap. If I have them sprint too early, before their bodies are sufficiently recovered, their sprints will turn into jogging. And jogging is fine, for aerobic work. Not when we're sprinting.

The third will probably strike close to home with many of you in some form or another, if you've spent any time in the gym or running. Have you ever tried to max out on a squat or deadlift (or run for a personal best in a race)? You rack more weight on the squat bar than you've ever had on before. You've been training long and hard for this moment. You slide under the bar, lift it up, step back, and take a deep breath. You descend slower than you'd like to because the weight is so much. You finally reach the bottom. Then you begin the ascent. You're pushing and pushing and pushing. The bar is moving slowly, but it's moving. It feels like an eternity. The entire lift down and up took eight, ten, fifteen seconds. Fifteen seconds of grueling fight. Every ounce of energy and fight in your body, but you did it. A week later you try to move the same weight, but you're not even close. But why? You did it before. You waited a week or ten days. Surely your muscles are healed. Probably, but your nervous system hasn't recovered. That lift was so physically taxing that your brain-body connection hasn't fully repaired itself. And it may not fully recover for two, three, four weeks.

If you're reading this, you're probably familiar with some form of the above examples, and you understand that there's a certain amount of time needed to recover for each of them. Certain conditions must be met. For the first, you'll need adequate protein and time for your muscles to rebuild on top of the broken-down muscle fibers. For the second, enough time between laps must be adequate for the body to restore glycogen and ATP back into the mitochondria of the cell. We understand the concept of recovery, but we don't necessarily understand how to identify any level of overtraining, or when we aren't fully recovered for the next similar training.

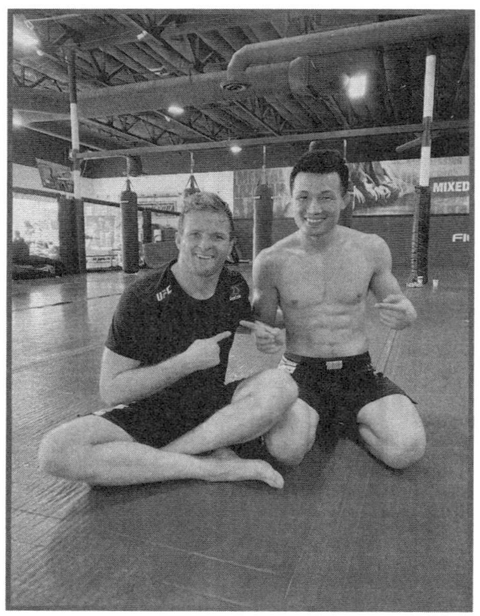

Zombie was so fatigued, but couldn't push his HR very high, which is the first sign of overtraining. We corrected and he went on to win a unanimous decision over the always tough Dan Ige.

Seigher Brown

EVERYWHERE WERE SIGNS

The most common symptoms of overtraining:

Plateauing heart rate: Falsely, people regularly relate a heart rate that won't increase into zone 4 or 5 as the sign of a healthy heart.

Before Korean Zombie fought Dan Ige, we were in a training session and Zombie was exhausted. He's a constantly overtrained athlete. He pushes and pushes and pushes. More is always better. It's a very "Asian" approach to MMA training—always go harder. We were trying to spike his heart rate, but his body was like a bowl of noodles. He and our striking coach conversed in Korean for a moment and then turned to me.

"Zombie doesn't know why he can't turn it up to that next gear. His heart rate isn't even high—it actually won't even go over 160, so he's gotta be in great shape, right?"

"Oh no. Let me see his phone," I said, and looked at the training session. It peaked at 161 bpm. "He's overtrained," I said.

"What? But his heart rate won't even get high."

"Yeah, that's one of the first signs."

Fortunately, Zombie went home and rested. We significantly decreased his workout volume for a few days and he recovered well. A few days later and he was back to his normal self, knocking out sparring partners one after the other. He won a unanimous decision over Dan Ige.

Trouble sleeping: This is usually the first symptom of overtraining. The moment a fighter tells me she can't sleep, I send her home. Go rest. There's nothing we can do here that's more important than you recovering and giving your body time to relax and rebuild. I've talked about sleep a lot. There's no need to speak further on it here, but just recognize trouble sleeping as a major red flag in the world of athletic overtraining/recovery.

Jump test: I don't use this much, but many college teams test vertical jump as a baseline. When an athlete's vertical jump decreases significantly from its baseline, it's a major indicator of overtraining and lack of recovery.

Flu/cold/cold sores/infections: I'm not sure these would be "symptoms" of overtraining or a "response" to overtraining, but nonetheless, overtraining will significantly hinder your immune system, and I've seen countless fighters bedridden from cold or flu viruses mid-camp and breaking out with cold sores or herpes or even swallowing antibiotics due to staph infections.

The gold standard

Up until fairly recently, coaches and athletes had the "always go harder" attitude. You're tired? Push harder. You're sore? Push harder. You're slower? Push harder. Not catching the ball? More reps. Got hit too many times? More reps. More, more, more. Harder, harder, harder. Until you hit the overtrained wall. And then you're toast. Good luck. But over the last ten to twenty years, scientists have begun to put more into the study of sports science and recovery. There's a lot more money in it these days—there's a massive market in college and professional sports, but there's also a much, much bigger market too, in the weekend warrior and everyday person, who until recently smoked, ate more red meat, and drank a lot more. And with all of that, the market for wearable health tracking technology has exploded.

The wearable technology really started decades ago and was made popular most notably by the Polar company, which developed a wearable heart rate monitor that runners and swimmers could use to track their heart rate during exercise. Over the years, that technology has grown and seeped into other sports labs and onto the fields of numerous activities and morphed into hundreds of watches, straps, and apps—all tracking bio data that can be used to understand the body in ways we never thought possible. With all this newfound interest and technology, the science is showing that smarter, not harder really is the key to optimal performance. The days of "push through" every second of our athletic lives may be coming to an end. With our ability to track our HRV with a wristwatch, we know if we should go for that PR or if we should complete a slow aerobic jog. Did we get a great night's sleep where our body was able to fully recover, or are we going to crash as soon as our morning coffee wears off?

We could talk biometrics until we're blue in the face, and there are a ton of them being tracked by your Apple Watch, Garmin, Polar, and Oura Ring. Daily steps, body temperature, and blood oxygen levels are just a few, but there's only one I really care about in terms of recoverability, and that's HRV.

Heart rate variability (HRV) refers to the natural fluctuations in the time intervals between consecutive heartbeats. It is a measure of how well the autonomic nervous system (ANS), which controls involuntary bodily functions like heart rate, is functioning.

WHAT IS HEART RATE VARIABILITY?

HRV is typically measured in milliseconds (ms) using a heart rate monitor or electrocardiogram (ECG). The time intervals between heartbeats are calculated and then analyzed to determine the following parameters. Translation: In between our actual heartbeats we have a series of "micro" heartbeats. Those microbeats are what are being measured by our HRV wearable monitors.

Importance of HRV: Our HRV is an important indicator of overall cardiovascular health and autonomic nervous system function. A higher HRV generally indicates:

- **Better stress management: The ANS is able to adapt more effectively to changes in stress.**

- Improved cardiovascular health: Reduced risk of heart disease and other cardiovascular conditions.

- Enhanced athletic performance: The body is more efficient at recovering from exercise.

Each person's baseline HRV will vary by genetics, physiology, age, and the strength of each person's cardiovascular system, so my HRV of 50 might be amazing, where a 19-year-old competitive swimmer might have a baseline HRV of 80. By using a wearable monitor, you can track your HRV and build your own baseline, and then the algorithmic app will transfer that information into a "readiness" score for your daily activity, though some may use a different term than "readiness." HRV also helps us decide whether to work toward a PR on the weights or go for a brisk walk around the park.

Dr. Fomin of the UFC PI loves using HRV as well as self-reported readiness to track how prepared an athlete is for training, and at what intensity she should train at because he needs to know how "full or empty their tank is." I asked him why HRV matters and why is overtraining so bad?

"Athletes are limited to their 'training' gallons a day. Imagine if I told you to drink this glass of water. You drink it. No problem. But now I ask you to drink this gallon of water. Could you do it? Maybe. Maybe you could, but it would be very difficult. But now I have a 5-gallon tank of water and I ask you to drink that. You most certainly couldn't drink that all. That is your training load. There are only so many training gallons you can drink in a day. But unlike the water, excessive training gallons raise the level of toxicity in your body due to metabolic waste."

Dr. Fomin suggests a few simple strategies for managing workload and limiting overtraining:

First and foremost?

- **Stress dosage management: Time and again, I come back to managing load, not overdoing things, the holistic approach.**

- **Recovery > overload:** Athletes process limited "training gallons" daily—exceeding causes systemic inflammation. It's better to be 5% undertrained than 5% overtrained. Be recovered, and when you are fully recovered, push yourself to the absolute max, but don't try to push yourself when there's nothing left in the proverbial gas tank. Nothing but diminishing returns will occur.

- **Specialization hierarchy** (Dr. Fomin's recommended approach for MMA):
  MMA-specific training (70%+ of program).

Targeted S&C (compound lifts max intent [going to failure]).

Recovery modalities (contrast therapy, HRV-guided naps).

He also is adamant about reducing excess stimuli during fight week and says not to introduce any novel stimuli or exceed 85% max HR, and getting anything less than 9 hours of sleep a night is a definite "NO!" All of which will help ensure adequate HRV and readiness on fight day.

Santino's note on wearables and bio-tracking: Don't overdo it. I initially had planned to write a chapter dedicated to wearables and trackers for this book. I really do love the science behind all the bio data. The issue with the bio data is threefold.

First, and most importantly, once you begin to obsess over the data and it becomes its own source of stress, it's time to put the wearable away for a bit. When I first began tracking my bio data, I loved watching the way a single beer affected my sleep, or how timing my meals would change my deep sleep vs rem sleep. I loved staring at my readiness score after easy workouts and hard workouts and how the way I trained day after day and week after week affected my HRV, but eventually, I—and pretty much every fighter I've trained has done this at some point—allowed the bio data to dictate my life. I found myself staying awake at night worried that I ate too late and my sleep would be compromised. I found myself sitting out of training as I was in the orange today and was worried about being in the red zone tomorrow when I planned to run a hard 5 miles. Fighters do that too—they sit out of practice, skip practice, panic over metric and sleep data. I even remember Charles Stull, of the UFC PI, telling me, "Yeah, I pretty much stopped wearing my Oura Ring altogether. I started obsessing about it, and it became more detrimental than beneficial." I feel the same way at this point in my life. But I am glad I did wear it for years, as it really helped me understand my body and how I should periodize my training and prioritize sleep—which I always do! But now I have a better internal understanding and don't really need the numbers tracked day in and out.

The second note is that a lot of the wearables are inconsistent with their data, and I'm not sure I believe the accuracy of the readings. One week Kamuela and I had him wearing multiple bio data trackers and even purchased an Omegawave—at one point considered the gold standard of bio tracking—with its electrodes stuck all over the body like an EEG and EKG combined. We ran Kamuela into the ground with how hard we pushed every system we could think of, and all but the Polar said he was a 10/10 readiness for training every day. Day after day, we beat him down, and he was beyond exhausted—but numerous wearables told him he was fine. It's hard to trust "science" and "technology" when we see those results.

The last note, too much data isn't always usable. When we start introducing excess "noise" as Dr. Fomin calls it, many times all we do is confuse ourselves and cause anxiety. Just as with pretty much everything in this book, sometimes less is more.

WHEN IN DOUBT JUST REMEMBER THE 3 R'S

- **Rest: Get adequate rest between training sessions.**

- **Refuel:** Ensure protein and carbohydrates as quickly as possible after any workout. This will significantly improve your recovery, and help speed it up.

- **Rehydrate:** Drink, drink, drink! Being dehydrated results in a massive decline in physical abilities AND cognitive function.

PART THREE

Abs Are Made in the Kitchen

Diet and nutrition are both key contributing factors to fight readiness. So, too, is weight management. As both a former fighter and in my work as a trainer I have seen and participated in hundreds of weight cuts, some of which were brutal, not to mention dangerous. But diet, nutrition, and weight loss don't have to be the vicious cycles they so frequently are. We don't have to submit to fads or gimmicks or to the insecurities they shamelessly prey on. Much to the contrary, there's a way to lose weight and maintain that weight loss healthfully, sensibly, and in a way that even allows for some backsliding and an occasional cheat day.

For as complicated as we all make dieting, it's rather quite simple. It's not easy to adhere to, but it is simple. It's calories in versus calories out. Well, kind of. It's the right calories in at the right time versus the right amount of calories burned, whether by base metabolic rate (i.e., how many calories your body burns while at rest), or through exercise. It's not exciting, but it works.

Santino's note: I'm not a registered dietician, and I'm not trying to give you standard nutritional or medical advice here. This section is for people who want to lose weight. I'm not going to tell you how many grams of protein per kilogram of body weight is needed to add muscle (I will discuss protein in the next chapter, though) and I'm not going to discuss antioxidants and how they may be beneficial for your longevity. I'm not here to help you live longer through nutrition and, in actuality, if you are cutting extreme weight for extended periods of time, I'm probably going to help you die earlier than you otherwise would. My goal here is to get you on the scale as safely as possible, seeing the number you want to see—whether for sports performance or for your wedding photos. But if you are here for sports performance, I want you to perform well. I tell my fighters all the time, "Don't celebrate the scale. You didn't do anything yet, and making weight isn't an accomplishment. It's an entrance ticket. All it does is give you access to fight or wrestle or ride or whatever." Don't forget what the goal is—to win, not show up, and it drives me insane when people die to make the weight, only to leave all their fight behind on the scale. But if you just want to look good? I'm okay with that too!

12

NUTRITION FOR SPORTS PERFORMANCE

A WEIGHT CUT IS NOT A DIET, NOR IS IT PROPER NUTRITION

There are countless sports that require athletes to enter competitions as light as possible, while others are contested in specific weight classes that require people to weigh within a certain range, so participants may compete against others within the same weight range. Wrestlers, boxers, MMA fighters, weightlifters, and horse jockeys are just a few examples of sports that are heavily predicated upon large, drastic, weight cuts—which really brings us to the difference between a weight cut and keeping a naturally healthy walking around weight. And they are very different.

You might think the MMA athletes you see in the cage or the fitness competitors on stage keep their weight down yearlong, or, at least, season-long, but you'd be very mistaken. On average, most of my fighters come into camp about 20–30 lb. above the weight limit they will tip the scales at the day before their fight—when it's official. Some get as high as 50 lb. over their weight limit, while others are still 20 lb. overweight just a few days before they jump on the scale.

WHY LOSE WEIGHT? WHY NOT COMPETE IN YOUR NATURAL WEIGHT CLASS?

Combat sports' million-dollar question to every athlete is which weight class she should compete in. In MMA, let's look at a woman who walks around at 150 lb. out of camp—this is her training on a semiregular basis (4–5 practices a week), where she's probably running 1–2 times a week or lifting 1–2 times a week, while also attending MMA team practices a few days a week. To put that in perspective, she is probably training 5–8 hours a week, versus 16–25 hours a week (depending on the athlete) during her fight camp. From the weight classes she has to choose from (125 lb., 135 lb., or 145 lb.), she has to decide where she's going to have the best chance at becoming a champion.

At 150 lb. she is probably 18–24% body fat percentage, and she falls right in the middle of the lightweight division (for men). Unfortunately, that division doesn't exist for women in the UFC. So she is forced to, at a minimum, lose five pounds and fight smaller women in the 135–145-lb. weight limit as a Featherweight. But, in reality, that's not remotely realistic because she could diet for a few weeks and lose some weight and then get rid of some water weight and fight much smaller women who weigh in at under the 135 lb. division, right?

And then there's probably the actual weight class for this woman, which is Flyweight: 125 lb. maximum (126 lb. for a non-title fight). Why would a fighter compete against someone who weighs 150 lb. when she can fight someone who weighed in at 125 lb. (though come fight time that same woman will probably be close to 140 lb.)? A few pounds may not seem like a lot, but I assure you, it definitely is. But what may be even more of a competitive advantage is frame. What type of bone structure do you have? What type of frame do you have? What type of frame fighter do you excel against or have issues with? Some fighters may weigh 150 lb. and be 5′4″ tall, while others could be 6′ tall, and that is a majorly different fight.

More muscle generally means more strength. More height generally means more reach. All things considered, the bigger, stronger, more well-conditioned athlete usually wins. That's just part of athletic competition for combat sports. Athletes want a competitive advantage. Any competitive advantage—and being the biggest, strongest in the weight class—is a huge competitive advantage. Maybe worse, though, is being at a competitive disadvantage because an athlete isn't cutting weight and is competing against those infinitely larger than herself.

THE REALITY OF "DIETING"

I know we want to think if we go on the orange diet or the bacon diet or the ice cream diet, we'll lose all the weight we need, and to some extent, that's true. If you were to go on a "raw veggie only" diet for three weeks, you'd most likely lose a ton of weight. But let's think about that for a moment. How many calories are in raw veggies? Not a lot. And if you were to do nothing but that for three weeks (zero exercise or consumption of food), your calories in vs calories burned would heavily be tipped in the favor of weight loss.

The issues with that type of diet, and any type of diet, though, come down to balance and consistency. How long can the average person eat only raw veggies before they go off the rails? After three weeks of raw veggies, and seeing the 20-lb. reduction in body weight, most people are going to eat lasagna for two weeks straight and add that 20 lb. right back on, and probably a few more for good measure. Crash diets are a short-term solution to a long-term problem and are going to leave you with more negative effects than positive when the dust settles. Research from the *Journal of the International Society of Sports Nutrition* shows that crash diets can lead to:

- **20–30% reduction in metabolic rate (congrats, you've actually slowed your metabolism).**

- Significant loss of lean muscle mass (you're now weaker and "skinny fat").

- Decreased performance metrics (slower, weaker, and cognitively deficient).

- Hormonal disruptions that can last months (hormones trigger everything from metabolism to growth hormones to menstrual cycles—do you really want those problems?).

UNDERSTANDING THE FUNDAMENTALS

Whether you want to hear it or not, the basic equation for losing weight is calories in vs calories burned. That is just the way it is. WeightWatchers kind of had the right idea years ago, which basically gives points to certain meals or snacks. When you reach your daily points total, regardless of what the meals consisted of, you're done for the day. For example, say you are allowed 10 points for the day. Your eggs are 1 point. Your bacon is 2 points. Your three servings of veggies total 2 points and that brownie is 5 points—you're done for the day. Now, you could eat two brownies and be done for the day or ten servings of eggs. It doesn't matter, because it's a point total system, and once you max out, that's it.

Dr. Eric Helms, a PhD in exercise science and nutrition, reinforces this fundamental principle: "The hierarchy of importance for body composition change starts with energy balance. Without this foundation in place, no other nutritional strategies matter much." This aligns perfectly with what we see in combat sports, where athletes often focus on complex strategies while missing the basics.

THE SCIENCE BEHIND ENERGY BALANCE AND THE BASICS OF MACRONUTRIENTS

Before diving into specific weight management strategies, it's essential to understand the roles of different macronutrients in athletic performance. Carbohydrates, proteins, and fats each contribute uniquely to energy production, muscle function, and overall health.

Carbohydrates

Carbohydrates are the primary fuel source for athletes, especially during high-intensity exercise. They are broken down into glucose, which is stored as glycogen in the muscles and liver. Muscle glycogen is readily available for energy production, making it crucial for optimal performance.

Athletes should prioritize whole grains, fruits, and vegetables as sources of complex carbohydrates. These provide sustained energy release and essential nutrients. Refined carbohydrates, such as sugary drinks and processed foods, should be limited due to their rapid absorption and potential for energy crashes, as well as insulin spikes that can occur after consuming refined sugars, which triggers a fat storing mechanism in the body.

Protein

Protein is essential for building and repairing muscle tissue, which is particularly important for athletes engaged in strength training and those recovering from intense workouts. It also plays a role in hormone production and immune function. Protein should be consumed from multiple sources such as poultry, beef, pork, and fish. It's hard to find a "bad" protein, as long as it's not cooked in fats and oils.

Fat

While often demonized, fats are crucial for hormone production, cell membrane structure, and the absorption of fat-soluble vitamins. Fats also provide a concentrated source of energy, particularly important for endurance athletes. Fats are especially important during the last few days of a weight cut, when they act as the main source of energy as carbohydrates are limited/eliminated. Athletes should focus on consuming healthy fats, such as those found in olive oil, avocados, nuts, seeds, and fatty fish. Saturated and trans fats, found in processed foods and fried foods, should be limited.

The simple definitions above are critical for choosing the right types of carbohydrates, proteins, and fats, because not all calories are built the same. Although total calories in vs calories out will result in weight loss if operating in a deficit, some calories are just downright better than others (strawberries vs French fries). Charles Stull, lead performance dietitian at the UFC Performance Institute, emphasizes, "While total energy balance determines weight loss or gain, the source of those calories significantly impacts performance, recovery, and long-term success."

SIMPLE MATH: CALORIES IN VS CALORIES OUT

The healthy, smart way to lose weight is incrementally. Don't try to crash diet, because you won't last and you'll rebound—and wreak havoc on your body. I have a female fighter, Tracy Cortez, who has starved herself so badly to make weight during numerous weight cuts, they've turned into horrific, almost near-death (literally) experiences. Her body has undergone such damage and stress that major metabolic and hormonal issues have been caused, which, subsequently, makes it even harder to cut weight the very next fight. During her last weight cut, she cut her hair to shave off—literally—the last two ounces.

Dr. Louise Burke, leading sports nutrition researcher, explains: "The body's response to severe caloric restriction isn't just weight loss—it's a complex cascade of metabolic adaptations that can actually make long-term weight management harder." Tracy's body became severely anemic due to the strain of the starvation, coupled with the hard workload of an MMA fighter, with the intense weight cut of dropping 19 lb. of water in two days.

See, the body has a harder time burning fat when it's starved of oxygen, which iron transports. Remember, fat is burned during aerobic exercise, i.e., oxygen burning. Carbohydrates are anaerobic. The body breaks carbs down into sugars (glycogen), and glycogen stores create ATP that the body uses for short-term body movements—which, consequently, break down into lactic acid. But fat needs oxygen to burn and oxygen needs iron to be transported, and when you've become anemic because you've done it the "wrong" way for too many years, well, now you're reconsidering your entire career choice.

The equation

Calories in vs calories out is simple. You take your target weight loss goal (total number of pounds you need to lose), multiply that by 3600 (the approximate number of calories in a pound), and divide that by your target date (the number of days from now until then). So, if you want to lose 10 lb. in the next 30 days, it would look like this: $10 \times 3600 / 30 = 1200$.

You'd need to be in a 1200-calorie deficit for thirty days to reach your target goal of losing ten pounds.

That's the simple equation for weight loss. The details don't really matter. You could be more aggressive with the deficit and lose the weight faster, or you could loosen up the caloric restriction and reach your goal at a later date.

WHAT'S YOUR STARTING POINT?

Before you just start shaving calories off of your diet, you need to understand how many calories you're eating on a daily basis before your diet begins. This is actually pretty easy with modern technology—there are scores of apps out right now that allow you to take a quick picture of what you're eating and it banks it for you. Artificial Intelligence for counting calories seems to be more advanced than tracking HRV via wearables at this juncture. I'd suggest tracking your daily eating habits for at least 5 days, but 7–10 days is probably more realistic—taking into account the nights out with friends and that extra ice cream sundae while watching Sunday football.

EXERCISE IS THE REAL KEY

Calories in vs calories out is a heck of a lot easier with exercise—and it keeps you from being "skinny-fat." You know the people I'm talking about. They look skinny, but then take their shirt off and don't have a bit of muscle on their bodies. It's as if their bones are wrapped in marshmallows. They resemble Mr. Burns from the Simpsons. Nobody wants to be skinny-fat. Hell, I'd rather be fat-fat than skinny fat—but that's me.

Using the simple 10 lb. weight loss in a month, we calculated a daily caloric deficit of 1200 calories . . . but that's just with food. What if we are also on an exercise program and we're burning extra calories? That will significantly speed the process up, or even allow for more weight to be lost during the same period of time than just diet alone will account for—and you avoid being skinny-fat!

If your daily calorie reduction is 1200, you might decide to split that into 600 calories from food a day and 600 calories from exercise a day. Look at the chart below, and you'll see some hourly caloric burn rates from common exercises for a variety of different weights.

You might go to a local kickboxing gym and train for an hour or run for thirty minutes in the morning and jump rope for thirty minutes at night. Maybe you decide you actually want to reduce your daily intake of calories by 1000/day, but also work out an hour a day, leading to a 1600-calorie deficit a day. Now you're looking at losing 13.3 lb. in the same thirty-day period. The possibilities are endless.

Imagine what type of transformation you can undergo in a 30-, 60-, 90-day period? We're talking a couple of months! In less time than it takes for the sale of your new house to close, you can lose all the weight you want. Think of what you can do during a college semester of four months or an entire year!

ACTIVITY PER 30MIN	WEIGHT OF 125LB	WEIGHT OF 155LB	WEIGHT OF 185LB
Aerobics: Low Impact	165 kcal/hr	205 kcal/hr	244 kcal/hr
Running: 5 mph	240	298	355
Playing Volleyball	240	298	355
Bicycling: Vigorous	300	372	444
Kickboxing/MMA	300	372	444
Jumping Rope	300	372	444
Swimming: Vigorous	300	372	444
Running: 8 mph	375	465	555

It really is that easy. Make a few lifestyle changes consisting of a little bit of exercise and a little bit of caloric restriction (barring medical issues, that is), and you've got yourself a very attainable goal. Well, then, why is it so hard? Why do we have an obesity rate of nearly 40% in America if it's so easy?

If you're a fitness enthusiast, or someone just looking to lose a few pounds or wanting to fit in that dress, this next section doesn't necessarily pertain to you (go find the extreme weight cut guide my fighters undergo at the end of the book), but as an athlete, you're not finished. Diet is 50% of the weight loss goal; performance is the other 50%.

UNDERSTANDING ENERGY SYSTEMS AND PERFORMANCE

Dr. Andy Galpin, Professor of Kinesiology and expert in combat sports performance, explains the three primary energy systems that power athletic performance below—and why is this important? Because you need to understand that our nutrition, just like everything else in life, is all intertwined! When we starve ourselves or go on crazy crash or fad diets, we're not getting the proper types of energy we need for our nutrition. We're not bears, hibernating in the woods, surviving for weeks or months on our fat. How often are you hungry? Multiple times a day. We need constant nutritional replenishment, or we create imbalances. If we aren't eating any sugars: imbalance. If we aren't eating any complex carbs: imbalance. Eliminating fats: imbalance. And that's why calories in vs calories out is so important. It allows us to consume calories from many different sources (fats, sugars, cholesterol, sodium, EVERYTHING), but by design, it forces us into moderation. Don't eliminate foods. Eat pretty much everything from a variety of sources. Eliminate (unwanted) calories!

Look at the systems below and their source of energy and you'll see how much you'll want a variety of energy sources for your athletic endeavors.

1. **Phosphagen system (ATP-PC)**
   - Duration: 0–10 seconds
   - Used for: explosive movements, takedowns
   - Fuel source: stored ATP and creatine phosphate (food source: red meat, poultry, seafood)
   - Recovery time: 3–5 minutes
   - Critical for: initial burst in combinations, power moves

2. **Glycolytic system**
   - Duration: 10 seconds–2 minutes
   - Used for: high-intensity combinations, scrambles
   - Fuel source: muscle glycogen (food source: high-glycemic carbs such as sugars from fruits, white rice, breads)
   - Recovery time: 15–30 minutes
   - Essential for: extended exchanges, defensive scrambles

3. **Oxidative System**
   - Duration: 2+ minutes
   - Used for: overall fight endurance
   - Fuel source: fats and carbohydrates (food source, fats: almonds, avocado, eggs; complex carbs: whole grain bread, brown rice, sweet potato)
   - Recovery time: ongoing
   - Key for: fight longevity, recovery between rounds

The main breakdown of energy systems used in a 15–25 minute MMA fight is approximately:

- **40% aerobic system**
- 35% anaerobic glycolysis
- 25% ATP-PC system

There's not just one system in use, so why would you consume only one food source? We never want to eliminate entire sources of food—even cholesterol and simple sugars have their purpose in our bodies, and both have traditionally been the bogeymen of many American diets.

In addition to eating the right foods on a consistent basis, athletes also need to time their food correctly, on a consistent basis. Eating throughout the day is paramount to a healthy performance, and regardless of what our parents said, breakfast is not the most important meal of the day. All meals are important, and if you're a morning person and engaging in a vigorous workout first thing in the morning, the last thing you'll want to do is eat a full, heavy meal—unless you want everyone to know what you ate as it spews out all over their shoes.

Possibly the most important meal of them all isn't even a meal, though. One of the most important, and often overlooked and ignored nutritional concepts I see from athletes, is that their post-workout refuel usually doesn't occur until an hour or so after a workout, if it occurs at all. Many believe getting at least some simple carbs and some protein within a 15–30 minute window helps speed the recovery process.

This is such a debatable area of sports science, and you will see studies saying timing doesn't matter, while others say timing is critical. You're going to find literature on both sides. You're going to find literature that says you need 1.6 g protein per kg of body weight a day, while others say you need 2.2 g per kg. Again, it depends on the year and the article. So, if you feel like you're getting better gains while consuming a postexercise recovery drink, keep doing it. If you think you need more protein, go for it. Just make sure you're eating regular meals with a mix of carbs and proteins, which will ensure you have broken down carbs and proteins in your bloodstream so they are readily available for your body to use when needed. Skipping meals is the worst thing you can do, and regular meals are the 90% rule of sports nutrition, so how you mix and match the other 10% is probably not going to hurt you, regardless of what you decide!

THE PATH TO SUSTAINABLE WEIGHT MANAGEMENT

I know I'm a broken record at this point, but I'm trying to hammer the simple format into your heads: balance. Consistency will always beat passion in the long run. You need to be able to maintain a healthy diet with a blend of carbs, proteins, and fats—and the occasional dessert is just fine. It's making good choices on a CONSISTENT basis that leads to weight loss and keeping that weight off. Remember the 90% rule!

STARTING YOUR WEIGHT MANAGEMENT JOURNEY

Whether you're a fighter, an athlete of any sort, or just someone who wants to be healthier, let's talk a few easy, simple steps to reduce your caloric intake, whether you're counting your calories or not. First, and foremost, start slow. The tortoise won the race, not because he was faster, but because he was consistent. Slow and steady is the way to go. Cut one thing out, and then another, and then another. Remember we are a collection of our habits—our daily habits create who we are as a whole. We're not trying to crash diet here—we'll get to that later, I promise!

PRACTICAL TIPS FOR SUCCESS

Here are the starting points I give my fighters and regular students to implement into their diets to begin the weight-loss process (don't get that confused with the weight-cutting process, which we'll get to):

1. Start with cutting soda out of your diet. I know, personally, if I don't buy soda (6–12 packs) I will drink a LOT less. When I'm drinking soda regularly, I'll put 5–10 lb. on in a month. I can't keep soda in my fridge, as I'll drink an entire 12 pack in a 24-hour period. I do enjoy the occasional soda, though, and probably even drink more than I should. Harvard's School of Public Health shows that each daily serving of sugar-sweetened beverages is associated with:

- **0.6 kg weight gain per year.**
- 26% increased risk of developing type 2 diabetes.
- Significant decrease in athletic performance markers.
- Reduced recovery capacity.

   Drink carefully.
2. Choose mustard over mayonnaise and olive oil over butter when the option is there. Dr. Jose Antonio, CEO of the International Society of Sports Nutrition, explains: "The type of fats you consume can significantly impact inflammation and recovery. Omega-3-rich sources like olive oil provide benefits beyond simple calorie counting." Butter and mayonnaise, on the other hand, are virtually entirely made up of empty calories.
3. Save desserts for the weekends. It's okay to eat dessert, just not every day. Charles Stull from the UFC PI adds: "Strategic timing of higher-glycemic foods can actually benefit performance when properly planned around training sessions." Remember, don't eliminate, regulate.

4. Eat carbs as your side, not your main dish. Have you ever gone no/low carb? It's hell. I can barely last a day—but I have zero self-control during my post-MMA/wrestling life. I started wrestling at twelve years old and didn't enjoy a Thanksgiving until I quit fighting—wrestlers will understand the struggle of having to make weight Thanksgiving weekend every year. Remember, the body breaks down carbs and stores them as two main sources of energy: glycogen and fat. Glycogen stores are used for anaerobic, short-burst movements of the cells (sprinting, explosive movements), and pale in comparison to fat in terms of the body's storage levels. Mostly, though, excess carbs are converted to and stored as fat. When eating carbs, the less you consume equals less stored as fat! But feel free to eat them in small servings, and we need to eat them. But carbs are one of the easiest things to OVERconsume, especially in the form of pasta.
5. Limit deep-fried food. Deep-fried food tastes delicious, but let's face it, we know our daily dose of KFC or Popeye's chicken isn't going to slender out our midsections.
6. Load up on fruits and veggies. I mentioned the "raw veggie diet" earlier, and though I was just joking, I dare you to find a person who eats a ton of fruits and vegetables who is overweight. It won't happen. Eat your fruits and veggies before your main dish, and then consume the proteins/carbs. Also, fruit makes a great late-night snack when you need something sugary. Hell, add some peanut butter to those apple slices and you're even better off. The fat and protein in the peanut butter, combined with the fiber in the apple, help slow the excretion of insulin when the sugar from the apple hits your blood—and when insulin is released, your body wants

to store everything as fat. Bodybuilders often take insulin shots to help them put on weight—bad, scary idea because if you stop eating (stop ingesting the sugar needed to complement the insulin), you go into a diabetic coma—but you get the overall point. That said, a sugary snack combined with fiber/protein/fat is better for you than the sugary snack alone (lower glycemic index with the addition of fat/fiber/protein).

7. Use your judgment. You don't need to be a registered dietician to know the salmon dish is healthier than the chicken-fried steak. And if you choose the chicken/salmon/grilled/veggie/fruit choice more often than the steak/fried/carb/cheese/sugar-heavy dish, you're going to lose weight faster.
8. The real key is tipping the scales from "eating healthy every once in a while" to "eating unhealthy every once in a while." If you can do that, you're on the right track.

ADVANCED CONCEPTS IN ATHLETIC WEIGHT MANAGEMENT

Clint Wattenberg emphasizes: "The goal isn't just to make weight—it's to perform at your best while maintaining a healthy relationship with food and your body." We're teetering back and forth here between general nutritional tips and nutrition for athletic performance, but I'd hazard a guess that even those who think they just need the nutrition for athletic performance don't really know the general nutrition concepts either.

A CHEAT SHEET FOR STRATEGIC NUTRITION TIMING

I mentioned earlier about the timing of postworkout refueling, but on the next page is an even more comprehensive cheat sheet by Dr. Louise Burke from her research "fuel for the work required":

THE PSYCHOLOGY OF SUCCESS AND WEIGHT MANAGEMENT: WHY YOU'LL FAIL

Dr. James Clear's research on habit formation reveals that successful athletes share common psychological traits:

- **They focus on systems over goals.**
- They understand the compound effect of small choices.
- They embrace discomfort as a path to growth.
- They maintain identity-based habits.

PRE-TRAINING (2–3 HOURS BEFORE):	DURING TRAINING:	POST-TRAINING (WITHIN 30 MINUTES):
Moderate protein (20–30g)	Hydration with electrolytes	High-quality protein (25–40g)
Complex carbohydrates (40–60g)	Fast-acting carbs for sessions > 60 minutes	Fast-acting carbohydrates
Low fat	BCAAs for fasted training	Micronutrient-rich foods
Adequate hydration		Continued hydration

Success in anything is severely more reliant on consistency and habits over goals. There's a saying, "A goal without a plan is just a dream." I'd like to take that one step farther, though, and say that even with a plan, most people still fail. Why, though? Because we can't commit to building habits. We're too short-sighted and want things "now." We want immediate results, and we're so impatient, we rarely see things to the end. And then we live a life of luxury and comfort, but growth only comes through discomfort.

Success is nothing more than a mindset. Success is looking down at your feet and putting one foot in front of the other instead of looking over the horizon. I know that sounds lame and clichéd, but it's true. How many times have you thought of going back to school for a new degree, or applying for a new job, but the time to attain those degrees and careers seemed like an eternity? Four years?! I can't go back to school for that long. Six months of training? No way. But then the time passes, right? Four years passes by, and you think, "If I'd just started school back then, I'd be done by now and have a new job." Time passes regardless of what we do; we may as well take advantage of it.

As humans, we're also risk-averse. We don't like the unknown, and we'd rather deal with things we dislike—rather, hate!—than face the unknown. The uncomfortable. How many relationships have you been in that you wanted out of, but couldn't cut the cord? How many jobs? How many times have you looked in the mirror and wanted a new figure? A new haircut? A new image? But you didn't do anything about any of them, did you?

That is the same issue we face when thinking about a body transformation. Thinking about how hard it will be to make the food, to store the food. How hard it will be to wake up before work and get a run in, or how hot it will be in the Arizona sun at 6 PM, when you get off of work. We're human. We like comfort. We like schedules. We like patterns. It's the evolution of our species.

A CRACKHEAD WILL ALWAYS FIND MONEY FOR HIS DRUG

People will always find a way to pay for anything they want. They will find the time to go on that date or play that video game. They will always do what they want to do. Not what they "say" they want to do, but what they really want to do. Do you really want that new job or degree? Well, you watching Netflix and hanging out with friends says otherwise. Do you really want to pay down that credit card debt? Well, you spending every weekend at the club buying drinks says otherwise. We need to be honest with ourselves, and we need to prioritize what we really want—not what we say we want. A crack addict will find his drug. He's addicted. We know what he wants. If he has to steal, hurt someone, lie to a family member, ruin every relationship he has, he will find a way to get his drug. The difference between most of us and a crackhead, though, is at least the crackhead says what he actually wants. He's truthful about his deepest desires.

You need to truthfully decide if you want to lose weight, and if you're going to be disciplined enough to put the work in. Then you need to start slow—but just by starting, you're already taking ownership of your goals and working toward them. You're building your base. Your base of exercise knowledge: running vs hiking vs biking vs weight lifting—and everything in-between. You're building your base of physical ability: developing some aerobic cardio baseline, slowly developing muscular endurance and strength. In addition to building a physical baseline, you also need to develop a baseline of knowledge. Part of the hardship of undertaking a physical transformation (or accomplishing anything) is the lack of knowledge. What should you eat? What has more calories—pasta with red sauce or alfredo sauce? What exercises work my arms? Legs? Full body? What's an Olympic lift? Should I run in the morning or afternoon or night? Right now you may be intimidated by all that you need to learn about health and fitness, but start slow. Take your time. Don't get overwhelmed by what you don't know. And try not to get overwhelmed by all the information out there on the internet and social media. Just keep going, and if you mess up, it's okay. There's always tomorrow. One bad choice won't ruin your diet. It won't ruin your goal.

And be proud of yourself. Be proud of the dedication it takes for self-improvement. We want to be hard on ourselves. We want to stare back at the mirror and point out our flaws. We want to yell and cry and fall off the rails when we mess up. When we miss a workout or eat ice cream. But don't be hard on yourself. If you miss a workout or cheat on the diet, be a kid who fell off her bike—pick yourself up, brush off your knees, and get back on the bike like a big girl.

MY DIET

Well, maybe not *my* diet, but this is a diet I formulated years ago because one of my fighters was mid–weight cut, and he couldn't get through a workout. Erik, a 135-lb pro, had to lose 13 pounds for his upcoming fight and decided to test the no-carb waters. He lost 5 pounds over a weekend, but then his weight plateaued. At the same time, he was showing up to training looking like a ghost borrowed his soul. He couldn't wrestle or even drill for more than a few minutes without taking a knee or taking a break.

I'd finally had enough and wrote him an impromptu diet. I still use this as the "base" of my guys' diets now when they don't have their own dietician or meal prep company to work with.

Breakfast

Two hard-boiled eggs (150 calories)

¼–½ cup oatmeal (after cooked) with a teaspoon of honey and ¼ cup berries—depending on the weight and time frame we're dealing with (oatmeal: 120–240 calories; berries: 20–40 calories; honey: 21 calories)

Lunch

6 oz. of lean protein (steak: 460 calories, chicken: 407 calories, salmon: 354 calories)

No-carb veggie (50–150 calories)

Snack

½ cup almonds (414 calories)

½ cup berries (50 calories)

Dinner

6 oz. protein (350–450 calories)

No-carb veggie (50–150 calories)

½ cup cooked brown rice (120 calories)

This entire day's worth of food is approximately 1600 calories. This is a diet I'd give to someone four to six weeks out from their fight. As they get closer to the fight, I'd cut the ½ cup of almonds to ¼ cup. The oatmeal in the morning and the brown rice at night are generally replaced by fruit as the fight nears. Most people seem to have more energy when we switch from the oatmeal/rice to the fruit, even though there's more of a calorie deficit.

Notice how the diet plan is balanced. There's a blend of fats, carbs, and proteins. Lean meats and fruit and whole grain carbs. There's nothing groundbreaking about this diet—it's simple. And people can feel free to swap salmon for steak or chicken. Grill the meat or sear it with a low-fat/-calorie oil/spray. Simple.

13

VITAMINS AND SUPPLEMENTS

Vitamins and supplements are absolutely critical to athletic performance, and I want to give you a glossary of the supplements I advocate for.

Protein, of course, is huge. Glutamine is big. Branched-chain amino acids (BCAAs) are huge. And then, too, it is important to understand what happens when there's a deficiency in electrolytes and sodium, magnesium, calcium, and potassium. Sodium gets a bad rap because it's generally considered a bad thing. But we lose so much sodium during workouts. Just think about sodium and potassium, the way that they work in tandem together. Sodium is what makes your heart contract, and then potassium is what relaxes or expands it. Magnesium plays a vital role here, too. Sodium, potassium, and magnesium are what drive muscle contraction. When you have muscle cramping, that usually means you have a lack of sodium. And if you have Charlie horses, the recommendation is usually to take more magnesium, because it helps relax your muscles. So, understanding those things and understanding deficiencies in them is crucial.

Creatine, which has always been big among bodybuilders, has become big among mixed martial artists as well, and now the research is showing a link between creatine and brain health, which can be a game-changer for those engaging in contact sports like fighting, football, and ice hockey, where the risk of CTE is so high.

SANTINO'S LIST

I have to preface this entire section with: **I'm not sure of the efficacy of everything on this list, but I currently use, have used, or have my fighters use everything on this list.** I wanted to compile supplements and minerals that I have firsthand knowledge of. There are quite a few names on this that I have personally tried, and have felt little to zero benefit from, and I wouldn't push on anyone in terms of efficacy. Others, however, I'm a big proponent of.

- **My favorites are on this list in no order besides caffeine (I love coffee more than my children 28% of the time). Caffeine is always number one (but, personally, only in the form of coffee for me)**

- Coffee, L-tyrosine (main ingredient in 5-hour Energy), alpha-GPC (aids in cognition and alertness), creatine (numerous benefits, but I use it for cognition and brain function, not physical function), vitamin D (hormone regulation), oil of oregano (antiviral, antibacterial), zinc (immune boosting)

Performance-enhancing supplements

- **Creatine:** Creatine is a naturally occurring compound that helps the body produce energy. Studies support improved strength, power, and muscle mass. It's generally safe for most people, but some may experience gastrointestinal issues. I love creatine for brain cognition, especially if I know I'm not going to sleep much—recent studies laud creatine for sleep deprivation and brain function. If I take too much, though, I cramp. My entire body will cramp nonstop and I have to take a few days off. I cycle this.

- **Caffeine:** Caffeine is a stimulant that can improve alertness, focus, and endurance. It is generally safe in moderate doses, but excessive caffeine intake can cause anxiety, insomnia, and heart palpitations. Give me more. All day. Every day.

- **Beta-alanine:** Beta-alanine is an amino acid that helps buffer lactic acid buildup in muscles. Studies show beta-alanine supplementation can improve high-intensity exercise performance by aiding in lactic acid buffering—the burn of the workout is what stops us from continuing. This helps delay the "burn."

- **Nitrates:** Nitrates are compounds that can improve blood flow to muscles. L-arginine is one of the first types of "nitrates" to hit the market, as it's a vasodilator (expands blood vessels). The issue with L-arginine is it dissipates through the blood too quickly, which led to the introduction of L-arginine alpha-ketoglutarate, a slower-absorbing version. Beetroot is a common pre-workout supplement that acts as a vasodilator in the nitrate category. Nitrates are generally safe, but some people may experience headaches or dizziness.

Recovery supplements

- **Protein:** The gold standard of recovery. Try to get 1–2 grams of protein per pound of body weight. That's a "range," though; don't go too hard in the paint trying to get there.

- **Branched-chain amino acids (BCAAs):** BCAAs are essential amino acids that can help reduce muscle soreness and fatigue. The building blocks!

- **Glutamine:** Glutamine is an amino acid that plays a role in immune function and muscle recovery. So many studies show the efficacy of glutamine supplementation helping to reduce muscle soreness and fatigue.

- **Fadogia agrestis:** Traditionally used to increase testosterone levels. Limited scientific evidence to support this claim, but Dr. Huberman told me to take it, so I do. I also took Tribulis terrestris for years as well. I'm not sure either work.

Cognitive function and mood

- **L-tyrosine:** This amino acid is a precursor to dopamine and norepinephrine, which play a role in mood, focus, and stress response. Improves focus, mood, and cognitive function, especially during stress. I love L-tyrosine, and I've been taking it for years. Makes me alert, focused, and in a good mood. Think caffeine without the jitters, but if I take too much, I feel drugged and wide-eyed.

- **Alpha-GPC:** A choline compound that may enhance cognitive function and memory by increasing acetylcholine levels in the brain. Years ago I formulated a nootropic and one of the main ingredients was alpha-GPC. Some European countries prescribe it for various dementia patients. If I take it by itself (around 300–600 mg) I feel focused and energized.

- **Bacopa:** An herb used in traditional medicine that may improve memory and reduce anxiety. Here's another ingredient I used in my nootropic for cognition and focus. I don't feel its effects at an acute level, so I don't usually take it as a stand-alone.

- **L-theanine:** An amino acid found in green tea that may promote relaxation and improve focus. L-theanine was also in my nootropic, but I have to be careful not to take too much. I'm very sensitive to L-theanine, and even 40 mg of L-theanine makes me feel as if I'd taken a dose of gabapentin.

Immune function

- **Zinc:** Important for immune function, wound healing, and cell growth. If I get so much as a sniffle, I'm loading up on zinc and my other immune system compounds (oil of oregano, thyme, cinnamon).

- **Oil of oregano, cinnamon, and thyme extract:** I'm lumping these all together, but oil of oregano is my real go-to here. I use all in conjunction with one another when I am feeling sick, or my family is feeling sick. These have antimicrobial (viral, bacterial, fungal) properties and may support immune health. This cocktail might have literally saved my life when I was breaking out with staph infections regularly.

Vitamins and minerals

- **B12:** Essential for energy production, nerve function, and red blood cell formation. Deficiency is common, especially in vegetarians and vegans. Give me a vitamin B12 shot any day that I need some extra energy. But it leaves a weird taste in my mouth, even if injected.

- **B5 (pantothenic acid):** Involved in energy production and hormone synthesis. I have fighters take B5 while in the last few weeks of fight camp to help with energy and fat metabolism.

- **L-carnitine:** Plays a role in fat metabolism and energy production. See my notes on vitamin B5. Same but different. Helps with fat-burning as a fuel source instead of carbohydrates.

- **Magnesium:** Involved in muscle function, nerve function, and blood sugar control. I use magnesium all the time to help me with bloating if I am consuming too much salt—especially when I travel long distances. I also use it if I'm stiff and sore, as it's supposed to aid in muscle relaxation. Too much and it's a laxative, be warned.

- **Vitamin D:** Crucial for calcium absorption, bone health, immune function, and muscle function. Many people are deficient, especially those who live in areas with limited sun exposure, or who have darker skin. Athletes especially need adequate vitamin D for performance and recovery. I load up on vitamin D. I usually take 20,000 IU, 2× a day. Great for hormone function.

- **Iron:** Iron is essential for oxygen transport in the blood. Iron deficiency is common in athletes, especially female athletes. I do take iron, but I generally only take 50 mcg 2–4× a week, not daily. Definitely talk with your doctor before going on an iron supplement.

- **Electrolytes:** Electrolytes are minerals that help regulate fluid balance, muscle contractions, and nerve impulses. Athletes can lose electrolytes through sweat, so electrolyte supplementation may be beneficial, especially during prolonged exercise in hot environments. Electrolytes are so important for an athlete's function. I live in Arizona, where it's very hot and dry. We naturally sweat a ton during the summer months, and then add workouts on top of that and weight cutting, and the deficiency in electrolytes (sodium, calcium, magnesium) will leave you fatigued and unable to sleep well.

- **Omega 3, 6, 9:** Essential fatty acids that play a role in heart health, brain function, and inflammation. My father and all of his brothers died between the ages of fifty-four and sixty-five—all from heart-related issues. I take these to help my heart and cholesterol, and there are numerous recent studies that 2–3 grams daily can help aid against depression and anxiety, which much of my family suffers from.

- **Glycine, choline, and inositol:** I categorize these as one supplement, as they will usually be taken together. Glycine is an amino acid that may improve sleep quality and have anti-inflammatory properties, but I take it for the "supposed" cognitive functions. The same goes for choline and inositol, usually taken in tandem, as together they are said to be involved in cell membrane structure and neurotransmitter synthesis.

- **CoQ10:** An antioxidant that plays a role in energy production and has some merit behind it for cardiovascular health.

- **NAC (N-acetyl cysteine):** A precursor to glutathione, a powerful antioxidant. There are some preliminary studies that NAC can have an anti-aging effect, which is why I take this.

14

FAD DIETS, FASTING, AND OTHER THINGS TO AVOID

You might lose a bunch of weight on a juice only diet, or a raw diet, and possibly lose it quickly, but fad diets simply aren't sustainable over time. Instead of keeping the weight off, you're more likely to rebound and gain back all of that weight. In this chapter, I'll identify some of the popular fad diets, share some of my fighters' experiences with them, and demonstrate why they aren't sustainable. I'll also address the dreaded rebound and what you might be able to do to avoid it.

Keto is huge right now. Seems like everyone's doing keto. But no-carb, high-fat diets like keto (as most practice it) are essentially just a repackaged version of the Atkins Diet, which first hit bestseller lists more than fifty years ago. It's nothing new. Furthermore, few of the people who practice keto actually go into ketosis. It's really just no-carb.

Everybody wants to go no-carb because it delivers big results in a short amount of time—much of which are actually the reduction of glycogen in the muscle fibers, which carries approximately 3.5 grams of water with it for every gram of glycogen. But athletes cannot go no-carb and perform at a high level because they simply won't have the energy to do so. Tracy Cortez used to crash diet like that. She would starve herself or go no carb for weeks on end to make weight for a fight, and then she would rebound so badly after the fight that she'd be weighing forty, fifty pounds more than she did at the weigh-in. The weight fluctuations also wreaked havoc on Tracy hormonally. And if this is how an elite athlete's body responds to a no-carb diet, imagine what it might do to an ordinary person.

If your primary goal is to lose weight quickly, then fasting (or intermittent fasting, which is very popular these days) is fine as long as your meals are balanced in terms of calories in versus calories out. In reality, intermittent fasting is just a form of calories in vs calories out in a 24-hour period. Why does it work? Well, humans don't have discipline, and it's easier for most to skip meals for 20 hours than it is to stop eating after one portion. Intermittent fasting is just an absurd version of portion control, but we'll call it something different because it sells better.

But for sports? No. Do not fast. Do not eliminate carbs. Again it comes down to performance. All sports performance is going to be carb-based when it comes to energy, efficiency, and fuel. But between starving and no carbs, no carbs is better than nothing. Waking up and eating three eggs is better than waking up and eating nothing, but ideally a balanced meal is going to be the best. You really can't intermittent fast and expect to have good performance. That goes for physical as well as cognitive performance. I've noticed that it's harder for people on low- and no-carb diets to maintain focus and attention. When my athletes cut carbs out of their diet, we no longer do a 60–90-minute practice. Instead, we'll go for 20–30 minutes—short and sweet and high intensity—and get the heck out of there because after 20–30 minutes their brain turns to mush. Their body is mush. They're just dying on the ground, completely worthless.

You can't push yourself to your physical limits without the carbs. And you'll never actually get better aerobically, physically, or with your muscular endurance. You can't get your body in the shape you need it to be in without the carbs.

We're coming to the close of our lecture now, and it's time to touch base on some things (not mentioned here) that you might have heard on the internet, which can be a wonderful playground of misinformation. I originally had a list of fad diets that I was going to insert in the text, but I don't want to. This book isn't about knocking others, so much as it is teaching you how to live in balance. If you are educated, you'll be able to sniff out any "diet" and realize in two seconds that it's a "fad" style diet, meant to make money off of your short-term desire.

Remember, if a diet completely eliminates anything that makes you scratch your head, it's probably not a good diet to follow. If the diet introduces an absurd amount of something, it's probably a bad diet, and do not follow. But more so than anything, you shouldn't be following any fad diet anyway! You should be eating balanced, healthy meals on a regular basis, and then if you eat something with more sugar or fat today, it won't matter that much. Any real "diet" will just be a reduction in calories built with nutritional, balanced ingredients of proteins, fats, carbs, and vegetables.

Although I didn't want to rant about fad diets and give them space in my book, I did want to cover some nutritional myths that would best serve you all to know that they aren't real:

- **Myth: You need to carb-load the night before every workout.**
    - **Truth:** While carb-loading is beneficial for *endurance* events lasting over 90 minutes, it's unnecessary for most workouts.

- **Myth:** Dehydration isn't a big deal if you're not feeling thirsty.

- **Truth:** Thirst is a late indicator of dehydration. By the time you feel thirsty, you're already dehydrated. Drink consistently throughout the day, especially before, during, and after exercise. Learn to recognize early signs of dehydration like headache, fatigue, and dark urine.

- **Myth:** Sports drinks are always necessary during exercise.
  - **Truth:** Water is sufficient for most workouts under an hour. Outside of extreme running/marathon/Ironman events, sports drinks don't improve performance.

- **Myth:** You shouldn't drink water during exercise because it will cause cramps.
  - **Truth:** Dehydration is a major cause of muscle cramps. Drinking enough water is essential to prevent cramps. Electrolyte imbalances can also play a role, which sports drinks can help address in longer workouts.

TRAINING AND RECOVERY MYTHS

- **Myth: Lifting weights will make women bulky.**
  - **Truth:** Women don't have the same hormonal profile as men, so they won't develop large muscles from lifting weights in the same way. Hell, at this point, women *wish* this were true! I wish it were true. Everyone does. But, sadly, it isn't.

- **Myth:** Stretching before exercise prevents injuries.
  - **Truth:** Static stretching (holding a stretch for a period of time)

before exercise can actually *impair* performance and may not prevent injuries. Dynamic stretching (movements that mimic the activity you are about to do) is more beneficial before exercise. Static stretching is better suited for *after* exercise or on rest days.

- **Myth:** You shouldn't lift weights if you're sore.
  - **Truth:** While you shouldn't work through *pain*, some muscle soreness (DOMS) is normal after exercise. DOMS is a horrible indicator of recovery.

- **Myth:** More is always better when it comes to training.
  - **Truth:** Overtraining can lead to injuries, fatigue, and burnout. Rest and recovery are just as important as training. Your muscles grow and adapt during rest, not during exercise itself. We talked about this at length, but I wanted to reiterate the ridiculousness.

- **Myth:** You can target fat loss in specific areas by doing exercises that work those muscles. Remember when people used to wear those "waist trimmers"? Ha! I do too.
  - **Truth:** "Spot reduction" is a myth. You can't choose where your body loses fat. Fat loss occurs throughout the body as a whole.

- **Myth:** You have to "feel the burn" for a workout to be effective.
  - **Truth:** While some muscle fatigue is expected, you don't have to be in excruciating pain for a workout to be effective. Remember, the minimum effective dose is generally enough—especially in camp/season.

- **Myth:** Muscle turns into fat if you stop working out.
    - **Truth:** Muscle and fat are different tissues. Muscle doesn't turn into fat. If you stop working out, you may lose muscle mass, and if you're eating in a calorie surplus, you may gain fat, but one doesn't become the other.

- **Myth:** Fasted cardio burns more fat.

  Truth: While fasted cardio may slightly increase fat oxidation during exercise, it does not necessarily translate to greater overall fat loss. Fasted cardio has also been linked to elevated cortisol levels, which, as we spoke of earlier, aren't exactly what you're wanting to increase outside of the periods of sleep where you'll receive the greatest benefit—and who wants to train when they're starving anyway?

- **Myth:** Avoid eating before bed.

  Truth: This myth is not supported by scientific evidence. For years, bodybuilders have been known to wake up and eat in the middle of the night, or drink casein (milk) protein as it takes longer to break down, which helps keep the stomach full and supply muscles with nutrients.

- **Myth:** Athletes should avoid caffeine due to its diuretic effect.

  Truth: I don't care if this is true or not, I'm drinking my coffee. And while caffeine has a mild diuretic effect, it is minimal and does not significantly impact hydration status in athletes who consume it regularly. Also, the diuretic effect is acute (short in duration) and doesn't maintain over longer periods of time, so total hydration isn't affected in an overall 24-hour period.

- **Myth:** Creatine is bad for the kidneys.

  Reality: Research shows that creatine is safe for healthy athletes when used appropriately. Now, while creatine won't cause kidney damage, if you do have any sort of kidney damage or disease, you should consult a doctor before taking creatine, as it may be harmful.

PART FOUR

Hit the Ground Running (Sample Diets/Training Programs)

Every fighter is different, and so is every training camp. I custom tailor a training plan for each fighter that is specific to his or her individual fighting style, physical needs, particular strengths, and opponent. While the typical training camp will take six weeks, some camps are shorter and some are longer. Let's look at some of the real plans our team used to train several different fighters, both men and woman, in a range of weight classes. And because most readers aren't elite mixed martial artists, I'll show them how they can adapt these plans for their own training needs. You may not be Henry Cejudo, Kamuela Kirk, or Tracy Cortez, but that doesn't mean you can't train like them.

This fourth and final part of the book is where the rubber meets the road. You've put in all of your time and attention preparing. You've made weight and visualized the fight over and over in your mind. Now it's time to put it all together and execute on fight night. In this chapter I will walk readers through everything that goes on in the final days (and moments) before a fight and demonstrate, using real examples from my time both as a fighter and trainer, exactly what can happen when fight readiness meets opportunity.

I could only see her hand from underneath the towels. Wrapped tight like a cocoon, or a human burrito, she didn't move. I watched her body closely to see if her chest moved up and down. Was she breathing? I caught her brother's eye. Uncertainty covered his face. I inched over to her and moved a towel from her face and forehead. Her eyelids flickered. She didn't open them. Her hand fumbled around until she found my own—she squeezed and then motioned for me to get closer and then took my hand again. "I promise I won't quit. Just don't let me die," she whispered.

It's 10 PM on a Saturday night and you're watching a UFC fight card. The champ is ripped. Shredded. The fighters are sweating and bloody and with each punch and kick, you see the individual muscle striations push through the thin-looking skin. The bodies—real life posters on the wall at a doctor's office, showing where each muscle group sits. The champ explodes into a takedown and both fighters leave the floor as if jumping in unison. When the fight ends, the champ gets up and screams and every tendon, every muscle, every piece of physicality and athleticism accentuates. You want to look like that.

Twelve hours before you watched the physical altercation, the champ was getting a workout in—what fighters and coaches call a "shakeout." A fight day ritual skipped by few. The rationality behind the shakeout is multifaceted. It increases the heart rate and opens the lungs—making it much easier to warm up and get going later before the fight, when the actual pre-fight warm-up commences. The shakeout helps keep nerves and anxiety suppressed. Usually, a fighter is much more relaxed after the shakeout. Nerves are great for competition. They're a necessity. Too many nerves on fight day cause the oversecretion of adrenaline, which leads to the dreaded "adrenaline dump"—a competition fear. A killer of championships. But the less-talked-about purpose of the shakeout is to further the rehydration and recovery process that began approximately 24 hours earlier. The process that took 15 lb. of water weight out of the champ.

Twenty-four hours before the shakeout, the champ sat waiting to get on the scale for his official weigh-in. His resting heart rate was 130. The weight cut was brutal. His face is sucked in and his teeth protrude through his gums, almost through his lips. He resembles an Auschwitz survivor more than a professional athlete. His voice is soft, barely a whisper. His ears have plugged up and he hears everything as a loud muffle. His blood pressure is low. His trainer holds his arm and helps him up. The stagehands walk him to the scale, keeping a close eye on him and a hand on him in case he falls—easier to help catch him. The scale reads 170 lb. on the dot. He smiles and flexes for the cameras. He has brought his body as close to death as possible to make the weight and will now go through every effort to replenish himself for the next 36 hours before he performs unfathomable feats of athleticism at the pinnacle of combat sports. Nearly dead to apex predator in 36 hours. Ripped. Shredded. Physical peak performance.

The champ certainly doesn't actually weigh 170 lb. He touches that weight for a fleeting moment. Just twelve weeks earlier he weighed 210 lb.—maybe more. This is how he went from 210 lb. to 170 lb. in twelve weeks. How he went from 18% body fat to 8% body fat. All while training for a world title fight. How the human body can go from one extreme to the other.

Ready?

In every team sport I can think of, and almost any sport I can think of, there are seasons. There are start and stop dates. Athletes report to preseason "mini" camps and then the "optional" practices, which aren't really optional at all. Then training camps begin. The NFL and MLB have preseason games and spring training, respectively. Eventually, the regular season commences—the dates for all are set months, if not years, in advance. In any fighting sport, MMA, boxing, kickboxing, fighters may have 12 weeks' notice to a few hours' notice. Dan Ige, a Las Vegas resident, got the call just a few hours before fight time to take on Diego Lopes after his original opponent, Brian Ortega, couldn't make weight and had to pull out of the fight. Lopes, a rising star in the promotion, wanted to fight, the promotion wanted the fight—huge dollars were being lost otherwise. Dan Ige stepped in and saved the day. He lost in a unanimous decision, though he took the last round on all scorecards. Fighting is like skydiving—you just don't always know when you're going to take the jump.

15

SAMPLE 12-WEEK TRAINING CAMP

CAMP BEGINS

The standard camp is six to eight weeks long. Usually, for title fights, we've been given ten to twelve weeks' notice. I'm fortunate to have been involved with five title fight training camps—not nearly as many as some more prominent coaches, but most coaches don't ever run fight camps for championships, let alone five. The big difference between an 8-week camp and a 12-week camp is the base phase in the first three to four weeks. So many fighters travel and relax and gain weight after a fight. That first few weeks really allows a fighter to ease back into training with so much lower risk of injury than we see in an 8-week, 6-week, or 4-week camp. They slowly bring their cardio up and focus on muscular endurance with their lifts. Athletes can also sprint more during this phase, as they don't have to worry about quite as much recovery, as they aren't sparring five rounds twice a week, which is very taxing on the body, and more importantly, the nervous system.

For long camps, I like to see fighters attack more 400 m sprints on Saturdays, and more 30-second interval sprints on Tuesday. As camp goes on, and more MMA sparring comes into play, those days will become zone 2 aerobic days, as fighters will increase their live training sessions and sparring sessions, where they will find those high-range VO_2 pushes. We always want to cross-periodize our strength and conditioning with our MMA skills training too. The S&C schedule will go muscular endurance → strength → power/dynamic → where muscular endurance will create more atrophy and DOMS (delayed onset muscle soreness); strength is the middle, and power will create the least amount of DOMS and atrophy. Conversely, the MMA skills sessions will be more technical at the beginning, medium in the middle, and intense toward the last few weeks of camp. All camps will follow some version of this, except for a 4-week camp—that's just a sprint to the fight.

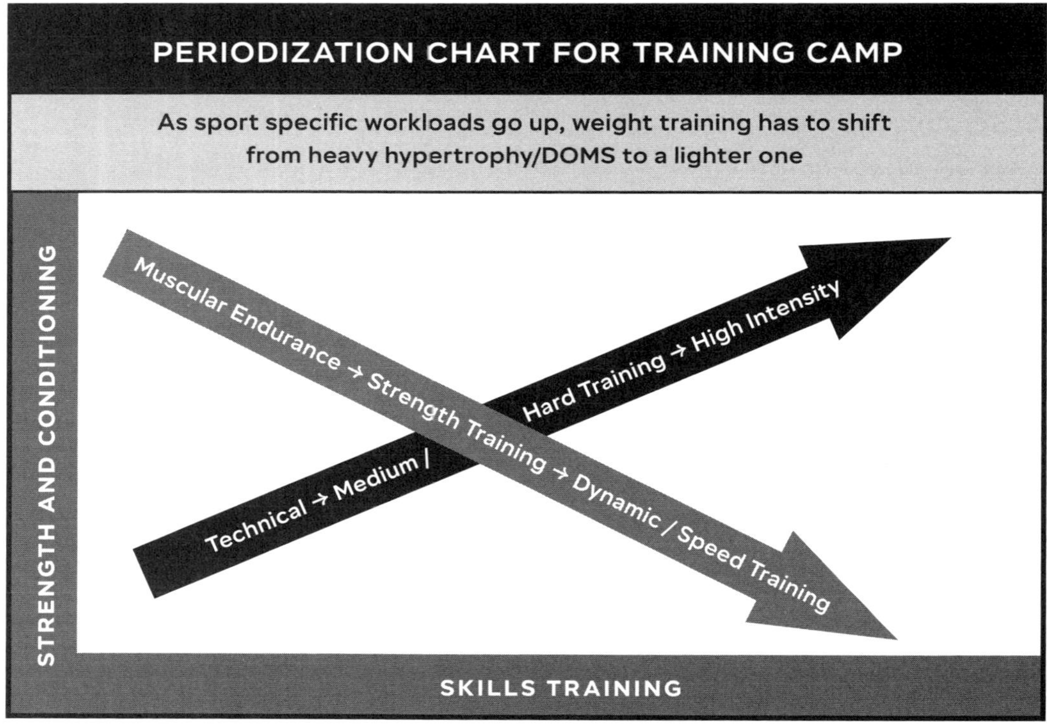

I want to use a few different scenarios for camps. The first, a 12-week training camp. Although rare, very important to understand. An 8-week training camp (assuming the athlete lifts weights out of camp), and a 4-week training camp, which really isn't much of a camp at all, and is actually barely over three weeks!

In terms of starting body weight and weight class: It doesn't actually matter because you now know how to calculate your weight loss. Remember, you can always calculate the calorie deficit you need to reach your goal by the following equation: Current weight – goal weight = total weight loss in pounds (191 – 166 = 24). Then we take our goal weight loss × 3600/days to our goal.

Our sample fighter walks around out of camp at 191 lb. and will be fighting at 156 lb. (non–title fight weight). When we calculate his goal weight, though, we don't use the scale weight as our goal. We use the number we expect him to start his weight cut from, as most fighters at the lightweight class will dehydrate out the last 10–12 lb. during the "weight cut." Remember, diet is for losing weight during camp. The weight cut begins fight week and ends with a brutally painful dehydration process called the water cut. For our fighter, he cuts weight well, so we're going to set our target weight at 168 lb. for the day before weigh-ins. Then we add on 3–5 lb. to be dropped from the time the fighter checks in to fight camp on the Tuesday of fight week, and we have our goal of 171 lb. So, we have 12 weeks to lose 20 lb. of actual weight, then he'll cut out carbs during fight week and severely restrict his eating and water load—we'll get to that in the weight cutting section. In 2026, May 2 is a Saturday. We'll call that "fight day." Our camp begins Feb 10—12 weeks out. We have 84 days until our fighter reports to fight week, which means we need a 900-calorie deficit a day to reach that goal.

This is where I need to generalize with you a bit because usually, between calorie deficit and exercise week to week and injuries and a random birthday, the daily deficit will be recalculated every week. If he's burning on average 500 calories a day more than we expected, we don't want him to stay the course, as he'll come in too light, and be drained of energy and increase the risk of injury. But if he's not losing the weight, we need to overcorrect and be more aggressive with the caloric deficit. We have fighters weigh in every Monday and Friday morning, so we know where their weight is at, and we can adjust. For this book and the examples, I'm not going to correct on a weekly basis, as everything is theoretical anyway, but I want you to have the knowledge to make adjustments to *your* training as needed.

Also, in terms of skills training, the first four to six weeks would really be a skills-building phase which we'd have identified during film sessions—we usually watch film weekly or biweekly for larger fight camps, especially title fight camps. I'm not going to go into a breakdown of each skills session. Those could be a million different things. And you might be applying this to a different sport! What I will do, though, is label the intensity of the workout 1–10 (10 being the most intense).

THE TRAINING

Diet: We will be operating at a deficit of 900 calories a day.

Skills training: This will consist of varying technical details, drilling, light live drilling, and sparring. Varying intensities.

Sparring: This is a variant of skills training, but this is also going to increase to max effort, very hard VO_2 max pushes. This should be the epitome of your cardio—it doesn't matter if it's zone 2 or VO_2 max or anything in between, you don't have a say, and it's just "your sport."

This should be the main source of all things S&C for your sport. That said, some people are injury-prone, and others may have injuries, so this high-intensity work can be supplemented by a vigorous mitt session or some type of circuit that suits MMA or your sport. For the purpose of this, we'll just call it MITTS on the calendar.

Cardio: One to two zone 2 sessions a week for our first few weeks, but then that will increase as camp continues; two VO_2 max sprint sessions a week, but that will be reduced as camp moves forward. The aerobic zone 2 sessions will comprise one 60 min session of running or stationary bike (labeled ZONE 2); the second will be a light mix of bag work and ground-and-pound drills for 45 min (labeled BAG WORK). The first VO_2 max session will be after sparring on Wed and will consist of 10–12 20-second max effort sprints on the treadmill (13–16 mph) followed by 1 minute of walking in between each sprint. The last sprint will always be to failure (run until you have to grab the handles and jump off—always assisted by coach) (labeled TREADMILL SPRINTS). The second VO_2 max day will be Saturday after sparring, which will consist of 3–4 400 m sprints. This will begin with 2–3 jogging laps, and then some dynamic movement prep. Fighters will sprint a 400 m lap, and should finish around 1:05–1:35 a lap, depending on gender, genetic speed, and athletic conditioning (labeled 400 m).

Plyometrics: This will consist of 10–15 minutes of plyometric work prior to the weight room workout.

Weight room: Muscular endurance phase.

- **Full body 2× per week (out of camp, this could be 3×–4× per week).**

- 1 set × 25 reps per muscle group (if athlete can only get 19 reps, lighten load; if athlete can get to 26 reps, add weight to load).

- All weight will be added based on number of reps, but should not significantly impact rep ranges.

- During the course of this phase, sets will be added.

First, let's look at the main lifts we're going to pull from all of our camps regardless of duration. The exercises are somewhat interchangeable (to a degree), so if you want to sub front squats for back squats or Zercher squats, go for it. Then when we go through different phases of our lifting, it's more about changing the weight and reps and velocity that gives us a different outcome, not necessarily (again, to a degree) the exercise movement. I just put the table on the next page there as a frame of reference, and you might substitute any number of exercises for the ones I chose. I wanted to keep everything as simple as possible because, in the end, it should be simple. The more we complicate things, the further we fall from our goal of spending more time in our sport.

But the single most important thing you can do while lifting weights is to maximize effort/intensity! If you leave reps in the tank, you aren't going to see the gains, regardless of what you are doing!

That said, during MMA camp, you do want to leave 1–2 reps in the tank, as taxing the nervous system to that degree will have diminishing returns during camp. Remember, the strength and conditioning is supplemental; keep the main thing the main thing. If you can't get your technical skills training in because you're so sore from the weight room, something's wrong. Now, out of camp, be as sore as you want and go get those PRs! Using out-of-camp time to make gains in cardio and strength is one of the best ways a fighter can spend time before camps start.

OUR MEDLEY OF EXERCISES TO CHOOSE FROM:					
Unweighted Plyos:	Weighted Plyos	Primary exercise groups	Leg accessory exercise	Bench accessory	Pull accessory
• Box Jump • Vertical Jump • Broad Jump	• DB Squat Jump • Barbell Squat Jump • Band Resisted Broad Jump • Med Ball Throws • MB Scoop Throw (for height or distance) • MB Chest Pass to Broad Jump	• Back Squat • Front Squat • Conventional Deadlift • Sumo Deadlift • Trap Bar Deadlift • Bench Press • Incline Bench Press Floor Clean Hang Clean • Strict Barbell Row • Weighted Pull Up	• Lunges • Split Squats • Zercher Squats • Wall Sits • Box Squats • Step-Ups • Straight Leg Deadlifts • Glute Thrusts	• Press Up • Incline Bench • Decline Bench • Dumbbell Press • Dumbbell Flies • Front Delt Raise	• Bicep Curls • Lat Pull-Downs • Seated Cable Rows • Negative Pull-Ups • Pull Upholds • Hammer Curls

WEEKS 12–9 (FOUR WEEKS)

Goal: strength base, aerobic base, VO_2 max spiking, skills acquisition

Week 1: 1 Set, **Week 2:** 1 Set, **Week 3:** 2 sets, **Week 4:** 2–3 sets.*

*Feel free to swap any of the exercises on the next page with the exercises listed above in the chart

Day 1: Compounds	Day 2: Isolated
Plyo Warm Up: 10 Min Upper Body Push: Bench Press Upper Body Pull: T Bar Rows Quads: Front Squats Hamstrings: Deadlifts Glutes: Glute Thrust	Plyo Warm Up: 10 Min Upper Body Push: Dumbbell Incline Bench Upper Body Pull: Lat Pull-downs Quads: Dumbbell Walking Lunges Hamstrings: Straightleg Dumbbell Deadlifts Glutes: Dumbbell Step Ups

Weeks 12–9 will look like this

FEBRUARY 2025						
Sunday	Monday	Tuesday	Wednesday	Thursday	Friday	Saturday
						1
2	3	4	5	6	7	8
9	10	11 -900 Start of Camp 9:00-10:30am Skills (6/10) 5:00-6:00pm Lift Day 1	12 -900 Start of Camp 9:00-10:30am Skills (4/10) 5:00-6:00pm (3/10) 6:15-7:00pm BAG WORK	13 -900 12:00pm Sparring (6-7/10) 5:00pm Treadmill Sprints	14 -900 10:00-11:30am (5/10) 6:15-7:00pm ZONE 2	15 -900 12:00pm Sparring (7/10) 3:00-4:00pm

WEEKS 8–5 (FOUR WEEKS)

Goal: Muscular strength, aerobic base continuation, VO_2 max spiking, skills implementation, and volume

Strength Sets/Reps: Begin with 65–80% of 1RM: **Week 1**: 2 Sets of 4–7 reps, **Week 2:** 2 Sets of 4–7 reps, **Week 3:** 2 sets 4–5 reps, **Week 4:** 2 sets of 3–4 reps (as the weight goes up, reps go down).

During this phase we're going to add in heavy sled pushes as well as farmer's carries. Both of these should end the workout.

Weeks 8–5 will look like this

FEBRUARY 2025						
Sunday	**Monday**	**Tuesday**	**Wednesday**	**Thursday**	**Friday**	**Saturday**
						1
2	3	4	5	6	7	8
9	10 -900 9:00-10:30am Skills (7/10) 5:00-6:00pm Lift Day 1	11 -900 9:00-10:30am Skills (4/10) 5:00-6:00 Skills (3/10) 6:15-7:00pm BAG WORK	12 -900 12:00pm Sparring (6-7/10) 5:00pm MITTS (Hard) 5x5min rounds	13 -900 9:00-10:30am Skills (7/10) 3:00-4:00pm Lift Day 2 5:00-6:00pm Skills (3-4/10)	14 -900 10:00-11:30am (4/10) 6:15-7:00pm ZONE 2	15 -900 12:00pm Sparring (7-8/10) 3:00-4:00pm

On the surface, this calendar looks very similar. The weight routine has changed (see above), the intensity levels have changed, and one of the sprint routines has been taken out. I took out the Wednesday sprints in case someone is prone to injury or happens to be injured. The athlete would have to lower the intensity of sparring, and then supplement that high-intensity work with something else (each athlete is different, and these are just examples of how you *might* program for a fighter). So often, schedules are merely guides, and daily adjustments have to be made to accommodate athletes. If we don't accommodate an athlete almost on a daily level, we may as well just send them off on their own and tell them to go to a CrossFit gym.

Another note on the intensity levels: As the intensity levels of sports training increase, the rep number with weights has to decrease. There are only so many minutes during the day an athlete can train, and unless we're all stabbing needles in our legs with steroids, an athlete must balance his load and reduce somewhere—remember, it's all about load management. If an athlete's S&C coach gets 100% out of him, well, that leaves 0% for any other work that day. The resources are finite.

WEEKS 4–1 (3.5 WEEKS)

Goal: maintaining strength, but shifting to power and speed (lower DOMS), maximizing VO_2 max, maximizing aerobic system, skills execution

Strength Sets/Reps: I see a lot of strength coaches really try to add weight here but keep reps to a minimum. I really don't care for that, and I'd like to see athletes using 65% of one rep max, but just throwing the weight for low reps. Bands really aid on this, as they allow for tension to be maintained through the whole range of motion without overloading the entire system with weight. We need to maintain our strength and power, and decrease the risk of overworking in the weight room during this phase.

During this phase, you'll notice more zone 2 cardio is added, and skills training days before sparring are significantly reduced. A rest evening is implemented on Fridays before sparring. During this last phase, we want a lot of intense VO_2 max pushes in the form of sparring, but we need to overcompensate the workload by reducing the training intensity the day before each sparring session (Tuesday and Saturday). We also reduce volume by giving Friday evening off.

Our last sparring day will be the Wednesday prior to fight week (10 days out). There's no need to risk a cut or injury so close to a fight. Light "play rounds" may occur on the Saturday where sparring would occur, or maybe a hard mitt session. Strength and conditioning will also be eliminated from the workload on the Monday prior to fight week. The body needs to conserve energy, as the athlete is usually much smaller than when camp began and her caloric deficit is really beginning to take a toll because the intensity of the workload has increased so much.

Day 1: Compounds	Day 2: Isolated
Plyo Warm Up: 10 Min Upper Body Push: Bench Press Upper Body Pull: T Bar Rows Quads: Front Squats Hamstrings: Deadlifts Glutes: Glute Thrust	Plyo Warm Up: 10 Min Upper Body Push: Dumbbell Incline Bench Upper Body Pull: Lat Pull Downs Quads: Dumbbell Walking Lunges Hamstrings: Straightleg Dumbbell Deadlifts Glutes: Dumbbell Step Ups

Weeks 4–1 will look like this

FEBRUARY 2025						
Sunday	Monday	Tuesday	Wednesday	Thursday	Friday	Saturday
						1
2	3	4	5	6	7	8
9	10 Start of Camp -900 9:00-10:30am Skills (8/10) 5:00-6:00pm Lift Day 1	11 -900 9:00-10:30am Skills (3/10) 5:00-6:00pm Skills (3/10) 6:15-7:00pm BAG WORK	12 -900 12:00pm Spar- ring (10/10) 5:00pm BAG WORK	13 -900 9:00-10:30am Skills (7/10) 3:00-4:00pm Lift Day 2 5:00-6:00pm Skills (3-4/10)	14 -900 10:00-11:30am (3/10)	15 -900 12:00pm Spar- ring (10/10) 3:00-4:45pm BAG WORK

16

SAMPLE FULL PLAN FOR 8 WEEKS

(Includes Nutrition, Strength/Conditioning, Sport-Specific Training)

You're not fighting for a title. Otherwise you'd probably have 12 weeks (unless someone got hurt, then you have 5 days!). But you're in shape and you've been running and lifting out of camp. This sounds like Tracy Cortez—she runs and lifts religiously out of camp and tends to lighten her skills/team training following fights, and then eases her way back into MMA training before signing a fight contract. You don't need a caloric breakdown because you already have that knowledge from the previous schedule.

In my ideal coaching world, an 8-week, or even 6-week camp is the perfect time frame—IF a fighter runs and lifts out of camp and trains on a regular basis (which isn't too difficult to find fighters who train this way). Again, IF I had my way, I think I would have fighters try to implement "out of camp" camps where they solely focused on strength and VO_2 max (of course they'd be training MMA skills as well, but their "focus" would be strength and VO_2 max). Then, when they started fight camp, we could do very simple power movements (like the last phase of the 12-week camp to maintain strength) and focus solely on cardio and skills acquisition, implementation, and execution. Unfortunately, it doesn't always work out that way . . . but I can dream!

So, let's quickly go through an 8-week camp—much of which will be similar to the 12-week camp, but with some subtle changes.

Most 8-week camps are going to consist of skills acquisitions on a technical level and cardio. It's really difficult to gain enough strength, speed, or power in this amount of time to be meaningful. If we were to make huge strides in 8 weeks with our bench press or squat records, it would mean our skills training and cardio were significantly hindered by the amount of time we'd be spending lifting weights and how sore we were from lifting weights. Not to mention how heavy we'd be from all the extra nutrition we'd need to put into our bodies to facilitate the muscle-building process.

We lift to maintain strength. We lift to maintain power. And we lift to help avoid injuries and for our muscular endurance while fighting. We're not looking for PRs; we're looking to avoid sliding backward too far.

If our team is accepting an 8-week fight, I'm assuming the athlete isn't completely coming off of the couch, but we still have to ensure the fighter doesn't go too hard too fast, which happens so, so often: Fighter trains in the gym and look great. Moves great. Submits training partners. Never gets tired. Accepts a fight. Gets excited. Goes too hard. Doesn't rest. Keeps training. Fighter is injured, or sick, or who knows, but it doesn't end well.

In terms of where our strength and conditioning begins, we're going to pick up right at the weight week mark of the 12-week camp, and our focus in the weight room will be the same, but our overall focus is going to be more on cardio than on VO_2 max pushes outside of sparring. Too much too soon without the proper buildup taxes the nervous system too much, and the risk for injury increases too much.

Goal: muscular strength, aerobic base continuation, VO_2 max spiking via sparring, skills implementation, and volume

Strength Sets/Reps: Begin with 65–80% of 1RM: **Week 1**: 2 Sets of 4–7 reps, **Week 2:** 2 Sets of 4–7 reps, **Week 3**: 2 sets 4–5 reps, **Week 4:** 2 sets of 3–4 reps (as the weight goes up, reps go down).

During this phase we're going to add in heavy sled pushes as well as farmer's carries. Both of these should end the workout.

Implementing springs here is doable, but I'd stick to the treadmill sprints, which are significantly less taxing on the hamstrings than the 400 m sprints. A better alternative is to use aerodyne sprints or the hard MITT sessions.

Day 1: Compounds	Day 2: Isolated
Plyo Warm Up: 10 Min	Plyo Warm Up: 10 Min
Upper Body Push: Bench Press	Upper Body Push: Dumbbell Incline Bench
Upper Body Pull: T Bar Rows	Upper Body Pull: Lat Pull Downs
Quads: Front Squats	Quads: Dumbbell Walking Lunges
Hamstrings: Deadlifts	Hamstrings: Straightleg Dumbbell Deadlifts
Sled Pushes And Pulls	Heavy Trap Bar Farmer's Walks

Each individual athlete will dictate the approach. Does she need to lose weight or is she weaker than her training partners? Are we at a huge technical disadvantage or an athletic one? In my years of coaching, when there's no time for "building bases" whether physical or technical, you attack cardio and get as many sparring rounds and as much live training in as possible, which will help both cardio and technique.

See page 286 for what Weeks 8–5 will look like

After the initial 4–5 weeks of training all focus is going to transfer to cardio and skills work. Treadmill sprints or aerodyne sprints after sparring will commence,

FEBRUARY 2025						
Sunday	Monday	Tuesday	Wednesday	Thursday	Friday	Saturday
						1
2	3	4	5	6	7	8
9	10 Start of Camp 9:00-10:30am Skills (8/10) 5:00-6:00pm Lift Day 1	11 9:00-10:30am Skills (3/10) 5:00-6:00pm Skills (3/10) 6:15-7:00pm ZONE 2	12 12:00pm Spar-ring (8/10) 5:00pm Treadmill Sprints	13 9:00-10:30am Skills (7/10) 3:00-4:00pm Lift Day 2 5:00-6:00pm Skills (3-4/10)	14 10:00-11:30am (5/10) 5:00-6:00pm ZONE 2	15 12:00pm Spar-ring (10/10) 3:00-3:45pm BAG WORK

and zone 2 cardio will be king. Mitt work will also increase. The last two to four weeks need to be intense during hard pushes, but they shouldn't be long in duration. Zone 2 is long in duration. Hard pushes should be short and sweet. Lifting will be dynamic, similar to the last phase of the 12-week camp.

See next page for what Weeks 4–1 will look like

Day 1: Compounds	Day 2: Isolated
Plyo Warm Up: 10 Min (Jumps, Ballistic Throws) Upper Body Push: Banded Bench Press Upper Body Pull: T Bar Rows Quads: Banded Back Squats Hamstrings: Deadlifts	Plyo Warm Up: 10 Min (Jumps, Ballistic Throws) Upper Body Push: Banded Bench Press Upper Body Pull: High Pulls Quads: Banded Back Squats Hamstrings: Banded Deadlifts

FEBRUARY 2025						
Sunday	Monday	Tuesday	Wednesday	Thursday	Friday	Saturday
						1
2	3	4	5	6	7	8
9	10 9:00-10:30am Skills (8/10) 4:00-5:00pm Skills (5/10) 5:00-6:00pm Lift Day 1	11 9:00-10:30am Skills (3/10) 5:00-6:00pm Skills (3/10) 6:15-7:00pm ZONE 2	12 12:00pm Sparring (8/10) Treadmill Sprints/ Aerodyne right after sparring 6:00 ZONE 2	13 9:00-10:30am Skills (7/10) 3:00-4:00pm Lift Day 2 5:00-6:00pm Skills (3-4/10)	14 10:00-11:30am (5/10)	15 12:00pm Sparring (10/10) 5:00-6:00 ZONE 2 Treadmill Sprints

17

SAMPLE FULL PLAN FOR 4 WEEKS

(Includes Nutrition, Strength/Conditioning, Sport-Specific Training)

A 4-week camp isn't even a camp. It's a sprint to the finish and we just hope we don't get hurt. The intensity really can't be too high or injury is bound to occur. The focus will always be cutting weight, which is great for our zone 2 cardio—and there will be a lot. Even sparring intensity can't elevate to the ranks we'd like it to because the risk of injury is too high. Our calories are most likely severely depleted, as we need to be very aggressive with our diet. We need to lift weights, but we can't risk injury or even the energy expenditure, as we could be running and burning fat while increasing our endurance during that time. This phase will look very similar to what you'd see an NFL running back performing in the weight room mid-season while he tries to stay explosive, and uninjured, but not wanting to push the envelope too far.

Goal: Injury prevention, muscle activation, aerobic cardio, fat loss/weight loss, energy efficiency while not becoming sick or injured

Strength Sets/Reps: Begin with 50–60% of 1RM: **Week 1**: 2 Sets of 3–5 reps, **Week 2:** 2 Sets of 3–5 reps, **Week 3:** 3 sets 3 reps, **Week 4:** Fight Week.

Day 1: Compounds	Day 2: Isolated
Plyo Warm Up: 10 min (Jumps, Ballistic throws) Upper Body Push: Banded Bench Press Upper Body Pull: High Pulls Quads: Banded Back Squats Hamstrings: Banded Deadlifts	Plyo Warm Up: 10 min (Jumps, Ballistic throws) Upper Body Push: Banded Bench Press Upper Body Pull: High Pulls Quads: Banded Back Squats Hamstrings: Banded Deadlifts

This entire short phase will look like this

FEBRUARY 2025						
Sunday	**Monday**	**Tuesday**	**Wednesday**	**Thursday**	**Friday**	**Saturday**
						1
2	3	4	5	6	7	8
9	10 9:00–10:30 AM Skills (6/10) 4:00–5:00 PM Skills (5/10) 5:00–6:00 PM Lift day 1	11 9:00–10:30 AM Skills (5/10) 5:00–6:00 PM Skills (3/10) 6:15–7:00 PM ZONE 2	12 12:00 PM Sparring (7–8/10) Treadmill sprints / Aerodyne right after sparring 6:00 PM ZONE 2	13 9:00–10:30 AM Skills (6–7/10) 3:00–4:00 PM Lift day 2 5:00–6:00 PM Skills (3–4/10)	14 10:00–11:30 AM (5/10) 5:00–6:00 PM ZONE 2	15 12:00 PM Spar- ring (7–8/10) Treadmill sprints

18

FIGHT WEEK AND THE WEIGHT CUT

Fight week actually starts before fight week. It begins the moment after the last sparring session occurs—usually the Wednesday before fight week actually takes place. From that point on, every focus is about making weight. Depending on how overweight the fighter is, carbohydrates are cut, or significantly reduced, after sparring, as the need for energy has, for the most part, dissipated. If the fighter is lighter, maybe she will wait until that Saturday, until after she performs a hard mitt session or similar.

A SPECIAL BREED

I arrived with Tracy on the Saturday before her fight. This fight week was different, it didn't begin on Tuesday—Tuesday was fight day. We arrived in Las Vegas on Saturday for Tracy's *Dana White's Tuesday Night Contender Series.* A new addition to UFC-produced programming, where Dana White "might" give a contract to a fighter if he or she impressed him enough. In the earlier seasons, contracts were not guaranteed. Since the early days, Dana has since been more lenient with handing them out.

Arriving at any UFC event means checking in with staff and stripping down for a weight check. The UFC wants to see how far away from your target weight you are when you arrive, so they're not surprised if there's a weight miss or someone goes to the hospital. The UFC hates surprises.

"Imma be heavy right now. I just water loaded a ton right before we got in here," Tracy said to the man checking her in.

The scale read "142."

"Whoa. That's quite a bit of weight you have to get rid of. You sure you're good?"

"Oh yeah. I'm probably more like 137 or 136—I just drank so much water on the plane and when we landed. I'll be fine. Trust me."

Tracy needed to weigh in at 126 lb. for her scheduled affair. If she missed weight, she wouldn't be eligible for the contract, regardless of how impressive her performance was. She hadn't been water-loading, but had actually spent time in the sauna before we flew to Vegas to ensure her check-weight was lower than her actual weight. This was heavier than she'd ever been before. She'd recently had some emotional things going on in her life. Her weight reflected the difficult emotional state.

When we got back up to the room, she drank water. Her brother, Junior, and I stared at each other. We knew we were in for one. Weigh-ins were scheduled for Monday between 9 AM and 11 AM. The UFC switched to morning weigh-ins after they banned the use of IVs for rehydration to allow the fighters more time to recover before fight time. Because of the early weigh-in time, most fighters will cut weight the evening before—usually beginning the process between 8 PM and 10 PM. Sunday night or afternoon would be standard.

"I know we usually start cutting tomorrow, but I'm gonna have to do a cut tonight to get some weight off. I'm going to try to get 6 lb. or 8 lb. off today, and then start early tomorrow afternoon for the rest."

We packed our bags and headed to the UFC Performance Institute. The UFC

PI is a fighter's Disneyland. Free smoothies, drinks, snacks. Workout rooms, strength and conditioning specialists, massage therapists and physical therapists—anything an athlete could possibly need to perform and recover to optimize athletic performance. *Contender Series* fighters were limited to the use of the weight cutting equipment, mats, and sauna—they weren't UFC fighters yet, and they wouldn't be treated as such. The uniforms given were unbranded. The gloves were unbranded. The bags were small and virtually disposable. I liked it. They had to earn their place in this magnificent structure reserved for such an elite few.

There we met the new addition to the UFC's nutrition and performance team, Charles Stull, a registered dietician and a competitive kickboxer. He came on board to lighten the load for Clint Wattenberg, the nutrition director at the time.

"Hey, nice to meet you guys," he said to the three of us and then turned to Tracy. "I'm excited for your fight. I can't wait to watch."

"I want to get on the treadmill and just walk. Maybe a light jog, but just sweat. I sweat so much more from working out than I do from the sauna," she told us, though I was worried as I knew any workload via exercise was going to tax her since we had so much weight to lose. But a fighter knows her body, and even if they don't, having a fighter in the right frame of mind is sometimes more important than being correct as a coach.

"What's your weight?" I asked.

"144," she said.

After the check scale, she drank quite a bit of water, so we expected her weight to be higher, but it was still such a shocking number to hear. To this day, I think she might have been even heavier but didn't want us to freak out more than we already were.

After we applied Sweet Sweat and sauna-suited her up, she began the workout. She spent exactly an hour on the treadmill before we started our sauna sessions. We didn't need a full session, as we knew she would drink some water and eat a little dinner. This was just the start of the marathon; we couldn't sprint too soon.

After checking her weight, she'd lost 4.5 lb. She'd broken 140 lb., a big milestone. We still had a long way to go, but 13.5 lb. was a much more manageable task than 18 lb. We went back to the hotel, where she sipped on a little water and ate some chicken and went to bed.

Most fighters "float" weight during the night. Often a fighter will go to sleep a pound over weight, or even two, and wake up on weight or even under. After Tracy drank the fluids and ate a little, we didn't expect much weight to go back on and hoped for a good night's "float." In the morning she woke up and stepped on the scale.

"139."

Nobody said anything. There was no need for us to reply. We all knew the task at hand.

We started the weight cut again at noon. The previous day's process was repeated. The walk/jog for an hour was harder this time. We checked her weight.

"135.5."

Back to the hotel for some rest and then we'd continue later.

At 6 PM we were back at the PI. Back in a sauna suit. Back on the treadmill.

"Are you sure you don't want to go right in the sauna?" I asked. "Your legs are going to be shot."

"No. I know my body!" she snapped. "I sweat better when I work it off."

"Okay."

After thirty minutes, she was exhausted, and she finally acquiesced. We walked to the sauna. We alternated sauna sessions with our cocoon wraps (wrapped in towels and blankets to keep sweating without being subjected to the direct heat of the sauna) for an hour or so. Ten minutes in. Ten minutes out. Five in. Five out. Twelve in. Five out. At this point, it just comes down to however long a fighter can stay in at a time. But she had stopped sweating. She's sitting in a 200-degree sauna and was as dry as a piece of cardboard.

"You stopped sweating. Let's check your weight."

"132.2."

"Shit!" I thought. We're so far away. "There's no way she's going to make this."

We went back to the hotel and she slept for an hour. It was almost 9 PM, and the plan was to sleep for an hour, regroup, and then get back at it.

At 10:30 PM, Junior walked into her room. Her face was angular, cheeks sucked in. Definitely not the facial/cheek structure she usually possesses.

"Let's try a hot bath here. We don't have a ton of time, and if you sweat, it'll cut down on the drive time back to the PI. They close at midnight anyway."

We applied Sweet Sweat and drew a bath. We helped carry her from the bed to the bathtub; she slid in like a dead fish. After ten minutes, beads formed around the edges of her temples and above her upper lip. Fifteen minutes passed and she said, "I'm not sweating enough in here. I need to go back to the sauna." She was sweating, but in a bath, it's sometimes hard to tell.

Back at the PI, she said, "131." And we lathered her with Sweet Sweat and we all climbed back in the sauna. I was sweating. Junior was sweating. Tracy wasn't.

"Let's get you on a bike and try to break a sweat, and then we'll come back in here and keep it going." We picked her up. She fumbled her feet forward. The sauna suit swished as we walked upstairs. In the hallway she stood taller. She didn't want the UFC or her opponent to see her struggling. On the bicycle, she broke down and cried. After a moment she wiped her face and shook her head.

"Coach, I ain't no pussy bitch. I'm gonna make the weight," and she sped up.

After a few minutes, she opened the cuff of her sauna suit top and sweat leaked out. Water from the gods. Forty-five minutes later, we climbed back in the sauna. Ten minutes later she lay on the floor. Her brother ran to the

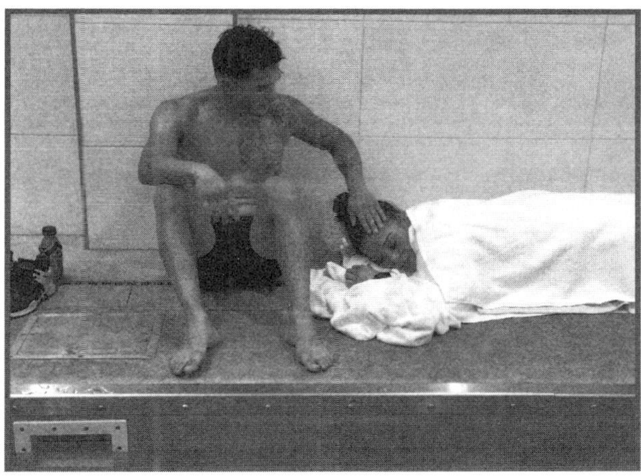

Cutting weight is scary. It's dangerous. And it should only be performed with experienced coaches who know how to identify problem signs that the cut is going wrong. *Seigher Brown*

bathroom. She motioned me over to her with her hand.

"What's up?" I asked. She grabbed my hand and squeezed it.

"I'll do whatever you say. I'll get in the sauna. Run. Whatever. I'll make the weight. Just don't let me die. Just don't let me die."

"I won't let you die. You're going to make the weight. You're going to win your fight. And you're going to get a UFC contract." Her back heaved up and down as she lay on her stomach as she cried.

"I'm done for the night. I'm not sweating anymore." We checked her weight. It was past midnight. Charles had held the PI open for us and let us stay until our session was done.

"129.4."

Five AM came too soon and Junior and I stumbled out of our room—hungover from our own weight loss and sleep deprivation—and knocked on her door.

We spent another session on the treadmill, but she couldn't stay on long. Twenty minutes of walking and we went back to the sauna, but she was sweating a good amount. She just didn't have the energy to keep walking. Sauna. Towels. Sauna. Towels. Bike. Sauna. Towels. Time was running out. We had to weigh in by 11, and if we were over, they'd give us another hour to cut the weight. If we weighed in at 9 AM, we'd have until 10 AM. If we weighed in at 10:59, we'd have until 11:59. If she stepped on the scale at 11:01, the fight was off. We had to get back and check her weight. We drove back to the hotel. Went to her room and began blow drying her hair. The UFC sent someone up from their crew to keep an eye on things. The UFC had been getting wind of the situation and were growing more uncomfortable with every person who came in contact with us.

"You have to get down there now and weigh in. The doctor wants to see you too. If you're not on, he'll determine if you can continue to cut," one of the workers told us.

She was over by 1.2 lb. Shit!

"Hey, Tracy, the doctor wants to see you," Charles said. She could barely stand. Barely walk. Barely talk.

She stood up and arched her back and stood straight up. Every last bit of energy she had in her soul she used to strut right to the doctor's room. She sat down in front of him.

"Hi Tracy, we just want to check to make sure you're still good to cut the rest of the weight. How are you feeling?"

She smiled, "Good. I feel good. I mean I'm cutting weight, so . . ."

"Yeah. I get that. Any headaches?"

"No." LIE

"Any backaches?"

"No." LIE

"Are you still sweating?"

"Oh, yeah. I just ran out of time." LIE

"I'm going to let you keep cutting, but we're going to keep an eye on you and send a paramedic to the room to make sure you're safe."

She walked out of the room, down the hall, and into the elevator. When the doors shut, she collapsed on the elevator floor.

She wasn't sweating and we didn't have time. We filled the bathtub and shut the bathroom door. It was humid. She had her plastics on and pummeled with her brother. We HAD to get her to break a sweat by moving. Heat alone wasn't going to work. She stood and pummeled for thirty minutes straight, but finally broke a sweat. When we saw the sweat, we threw her in the hot tub until 11:50. We dried her hair and walked back to the hotel lobby where the weigh-ins were being held.

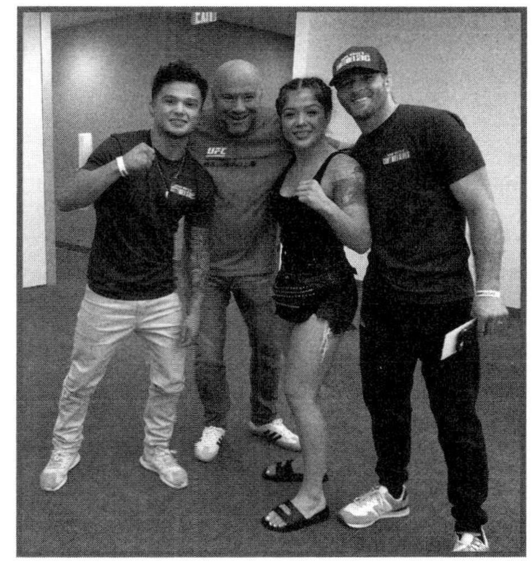

When you put everything into something, you get everything out of it. *Seigher Brown*

She stepped on the scale and we all held our breath. "One twenty-six!" the commissioner yelled. The entire room erupted in cheers. I breathed.

Tracy grabbed a rehydration drink from Charles and chugged it. They gave us a private room to sit in for a bit to rehydrate before we finished the check-in process with the commission.

She sat down on a chair and we shut the door.

Her body trembled and tears trickled down her face. "It hurts. It all hurts. Everything hurts." I've never seen anyone in pain like that through a weight cut. I'd never seen anyone endure a weight cut like that. I've never seen any form of strength and fortitude like that in a human. Ever. Should I have stopped the weight cut? Probably. Am I a bad coach for allowing her to go through that? Probably. Could she have died or been seriously injured by the cut? Probably.

But I didn't stop the cut. Tracy didn't stop cutting. And she made weight. She won her fight. And she received a UFC contract.

I said earlier that I wouldn't recommend anyone doing this. None of it. Not weight cutting. Not MMA. Not boxing. None of it. It's dangerous. It's all dangerous. And we know that, but we do it anyway.

Here's the fight week timeline for weight cutting

- **Wednesday or Saturday prior to fight week, carbohydrates are eliminated.**
- Saturday: water-loading begins. Consumption of 1.5–2 gallons of water is consumed a day.
- Sunday–Mon: fiber-loading occurs.
- Monday: Elimination of sodium from diet.
- Tuesday morning/afternoon: Fiber load ends.
- Tuesday: UFC check-in and weight check.
- Tuesday afternoon/evening: MiraLax/laxative to clean fiber and subsequent colon waste out of body.
- Tuesday–Thursday: The UFC Performance Institute takes over all meals and nutrition, usually resulting in a further reduction in calories, though not always.
- Thursday morning (the morning of the weight cut): Wake up and eat fatty foods—eggs, avocado, etc.—that are light in overall weight, but have fats to use for energy.

Consume 1–3 liters of water as quickly as possible when waking up—generally finished by noon to continue the dehydration process brought on by the hormonal result of consuming too much water.

- Thursday evening: Begin weight cut.

By this time, most people have already urinated out quite a bit of water and are anywhere between 7–15 lb. above their weigh-in weight. We usually begin by applying Sweet Sweat, a descendant of Albolene, a makeup remover, that helps to clean the pores. It aids in the weight cut, as it helps keep the pores open, which leads to significantly more fluid loss via sweat. Then the fighter pulls on a sauna suit (pants and top) to trap their body heat. I like to work off the first session of weight if I know we have a lot of weight to lose and it's going to be very difficult. We have intramuscular fluid and extramuscular fluid. Intra is the fluid stored in your muscles. Extra is stored in your skin and blood. By working out first, this (is believed) to help the muscles push fluid out prior to the heat exposure. If we perform heat exposure first, and there's still too much weight to lose, usually it's really difficult to motivate the exhausted fighter to run or shadowbox or ride a bike. However, early in the process, a fighter has more energy and can work the weight off. Maybe it's an overall energy issue (after an hour of sweating regardless of how she sweated, anyone would be tired), or maybe there's merit to it—I don't know. Cutting weight is anecdotal. It's witchcraft, not science. Science wouldn't put people's lives at risk for the sake of making weight.

Once on the treadmill, we don't run. We jog for five minutes at around 5 miles an hour (give or take a few for stride) and then once the fighter begins to sweat, the mph is reduced to a brisk speed walk. 3–5 minutes walking, 1 minute jogging. Sweating is the goal, not expending energy, and our bodies aren't faucets—we can't open them up and expect water to just flow from our pores. It's a long, slow process.

After 45–60 min on the treadmill, we either hit the sauna or bath. I prefer the bath, myself and for the fighters—others will only go in the sauna (air or blanket). I equate the sources of heat to cooking food. A bath is like boiling a lobster. A blanket is like a panini sandwich maker. A sauna is like an air fryer. Pick your death.

The bath needs to be hot, but not too hot. Again, humans aren't faucets, and if the bath is too hot, the body goes into shock and won't sweat at the optimal rate. Also, and if you ever try this, **this is the sentence that will save your life: it's not dehydration that sends people to the hospital and causes illness and even death, it's heat exposure/stroke.** Overheating is the real danger of weight cutting, not dehydration. Now, dehydrating yourself this much isn't healthy, but there are levels to dangerous, and heat stroke is by far more nefarious.

The bath should be between 107–110 degrees. Those temperatures are what we found to be most tolerable, yet produce the greatest sweat rate among fighters. Once in the bathtub, a timer is set when the fighter begins to sweat: 20 minutes.

When the timer goes off, we quickly help her out of the tub and pat dry the fighter. Another quick layer of Sweet Sweat is then reapplied and then the sauna suit is put back on. We then wrap her in towels/blankets for another 20 minutes to continue the sweating process, but with less heat than the tub—the tub or heated sauna can only be sustained for so long before people become claustrophobic. Generally, after the treadmill, and the bath, and the sauna, a fighter has lost anywhere between 3–8 lb. Women don't sweat nearly as much as men.

This entire process is usually repeated two, three, or four times—depending on the weight needed to be lost and how well a fighter sweats. With Tracy Cortez and Kelvin Gastelum, we've repeated this process for twenty-plus, thirty-plus hours in a row—with breaks in between sessions, of course.

ACKNOWLEDGMENTS

I want to thank

Dave Zowine for trusting me to coach athletes at his gym, and giving me the opportunity I needed to showcase my coaching abilities at a high level.

Eddie Cha, Angel Cejudo, and Alan Viers—all coaches who work with me every day. You've all taught me so much.

"The Glute Guy" Bret Contreras, who helped me early in my quest to find some answers to the sports performance questions that helped me find my "aha" moment when considering strength and conditioning in MMA. And thank you, Bret, for the interviews and the knowledge—you've always supported me.

Dr. Mike Israetel, for allowing me to interview you and pick your brain.

Dr. Roman Fomin of the UFC Performance Institute. You have given me more knowledge of the human body than I can possibly fathom. You're a genius in all things sports performance and recovery.

NOTES

CHAPTER 2: SLEEP IS A SUPER DRUG

20 Having one bad night of sleep: S. Garbarino et al., "Role of sleep deprivation in immune-related disease risk and outcomes," *Communications Biology*, vol. 4, no. 1, Nov. 2021, https://doi.org/10.1038/s42003-021-02825–4.

20 Sleep—or lack thereof: Garbarino et al., "Role of sleep deprivation."

20 In addition to physical ailments: Garbarino et al., "Role of sleep deprivation."

21 Early humans acknowledged sleep: D. C. Rosenberg, "A Look Back at the History of Sleep Research" | Blog | Sleep Health Solutions, *https://www.sleephealthsolutionsohio.com/*, Apr. 22, 2019, https://www.sleephealthsolutionsohio.com/blog/history-of-sleep-research.

21 In about 400 BC: L. Thomas, "History of Sleep," *News-Medical.net*, Aug. 23, 2018, https://www.news-medical.net/health/History-of-Sleep.aspx.

22 It wasn't until thousands: Rosenberg, "A Look Back."

22 history of sleep study: Rosenberg, "A Look Back."

24 Babies sleep a lot: National Sleep Foundation, "How Much Sleep Do You Really Need?," National Sleep Foundation, Oct. 01, 2020, https://www.thensf.org/how-many-hours-of-sleep-do-you-really-need/.

27 Overall, people spend: S. R. Benbadis, "Normal Sleep EEG: Overview, Stage I Sleep, Stage II Sleep," *eMedicine*, Apr. 2020, https://emedicine.medscape.com/article/1140322-overview.

28 But all of these habits can lead: K. Cherry, "The 4 Stages of Sleep (NREM and REM Sleep Cycles)," *Verywell Health*, Jun. 16, 2023, https://www.verywellhealth.com/the-four-stages-of-sleep-2795920.

28 When you come: L. L. Lewis, "All About Sleep Stage 2: Light Sleep," *Sleep.com*, Apr. 27, 2023, https://www.sleep.com/sleep-health/light-sleep.

31 Leptin and ghrelin: "The Sleep Effect—How Your Nightly Zzzs Affect Your Health," Communitymedical.org, Nov. 07, 2017, https://www.communitymedical.org/about-us/newsroom/the-sleep-effect-%E2%80%93-how-your-nightly-zzzs-affect-yo.

31 Ghrelin gives the body: "The Sleep Effect."

32 What we do know about REM sleep: A. K. Patel et al., "Physiology, Sleep Stages," *National Library of Medicine*, Jan. 26, 2024, https://www.ncbi.nlm.nih.gov/books/NBK526132/.

33 You're not here for a sleep education: National Heart, Lung, and Blood Institute, "What Are Sleep Deprivation and Deficiency?," *National Heart, Lung, and Blood Institute*, Mar. 24, 2022, https://www.nhlbi.nih.gov/health/sleep-deprivation.

CHAPTER 3: TECHNIQUE IS CRITICAL

72 Free-throw shooting before and after: "Improvement strategies in free-throw shooting and grip-strength tasks," PubMed, National Library of Medicine, accessed August 11, 2025. https://pubmed.ncbi.nlm.nih.gov/10843257/.

72 Colleagues tested video-based visualization: "The effect of Visualization Exercise through Video Media on Increasing Basketball Free Throw Shooting," *International Journal of Multidisciplinary Research and Analysis,* accessed August 11, 2025, https://ijmra.in/v5i8/8.php.

72 At the elite level of basketball: "Selective Efficacy of Static and Dynamic Imagery in Different States of Physical Fatigue," PLOS One, https://journals.plos.org/plosone/article?id=10.1371%2Fjournal.pone.0149654.

CHAPTER 4: PREPARATION LEADS TO SUCCESS

85–86 Preparation is addictive.: Tom Coughlin, *Earn the Right to Win: How Success in Any Field Starts with Superior Preparation.* (New York: Penguin Publishing Group, 2013).

NOTES

CHAPTER 5: HOW TO HANDLE INJURIES AND SETBACKS

108 Enhancement of athletic performance: "Proprioceptive Training Can Reduce Injuries by 50%," *Journal of Athletic Training*, accessed May 13, 2025, https://www.athletictraining.org/.

108 Reduction of injury risk: O. Yılmaz et al., "Effects of proprioceptive training on sports performance: a systematic review," *BMC sports science, medicine & rehabilitation*, vol. 16, no. 1, Jul. 2024, https://doi.org/10.1186/s13102-024-00936-z.

109 Preventative effects: A. M. C. van Beijsterveldt et al., "Effectiveness of an injury prevention programme for adult male amateur soccer players: a cluster-randomised controlled trial," *British Journal of Sports Medicine*, vol. 46, no. 16, pp. 1114–1118, Aug. 2012, https://doi.org/10.1136/bjsports-2012–091277.

109 Injury–risk relationship: J. B. Lauersen et al., "Strength training as superior, dose-dependent and safe prevention of acute and overuse sports injuries: a systematic review, qualitative analysis and meta-analysis," *British Journal of Sports Medicine*, vol. 52, no. 24, pp. 1557–1563, Aug. 2018, https://doi.org/10.1136/bjsports-2018–099078.

111 Effectiveness in injury prevention: van Beijsterveldt et al., "Effectiveness of an injury prevention."

112 Importance of gradual progression: T. J. Gabbett, "The training–injury prevention paradox: should athletes be training smarter *and* harder?," *British Journal of Sports Medicine*, vol. 50, no. 5, pp. 273–280, Jan. 2016, https://doi.org/10.1136/bjsports-2015–095788.

114 Proper nutrition and hydration: "Sports Medicine Research: In the Lab & in the Field | Sports Med Res," *Sports Medicine Research*, https://www.sportsmedres.org/.

115 Athletes wearing protective: A. S. McIntosh, "Risk compensation, motivation, injuries, and biomechanics in competitive sport," *British Journal of Sports Medicine*, vol. 39, no. 1, pp. 2–3, Jan. 2005, https://doi.org/10.1136/bjsm.2004.016188.

119 "We were in life-saving mode now": https://www.washingtonpost.com/sports/2020/08/17/alex-smiths-physician-feared-his-life-now-she-is-confident-he-can-play-football-again/

CHAPTER 11: RECOVERY

224 Heart rate variability (HRV): F. Shaffer and J. P. Ginsberg, "An Overview of Heart Rate Variability Metrics and Norms," *Frontiers in Public Health,* vol. 5, no. 258, Sep. 2017, https://doi.org/10.3389/fpubh.2017.00258.

225 HRV is typically: Z. German-Sallo, "Wavelet Transform-based HRV Analysis," *Procedia Technology*, vol. 12, pp. 105–111, 2014, https://doi.org/10.1016/j.protcy.2013.12.462.

225 Our HRV is an important: Shaffer and Ginsberg, "An Overview of Heart Rate."

CHAPTER 12: NUTRITION FOR SPORTS PERFORMANCE

235 Carbohydrates are the primary: L. K. Purcell, "Sport nutrition for young athletes," *Paediatrics & Child Health*, vol. 18, no. 4, pp. 200–5, Apr. 2013, https://doi.org/10.1093/pch/18.4.200.

235 Athletes should prioritize: D. Preiato, "Everything You Need to Know About Sports Nutrition," Healthline, Feb. 3, 2023. https://www.healthline.com/nutrition/sports-nutrition.

235 Protein is essential: Purcell, "Sport nutrition."

236 While often demonized: Purcell, "Sport nutrition."

INDEX

INDEX

INDEX

ABOUT THE AUTHOR

As a fighter and then a coach, **Santino DeFranco** has spent over twenty-five years honing his craft in mixed martial arts. He coaches MMA fighters at the highest level, including UFC two-division champion Henry Cejudo, The Korean Zombie, Kelvin Gastelum, and Tracy Cortez, among others.

Outside of coaching, Santino owns multiple businesses and hosts a weekly MMA podcast. He is married and has two smart, active sons.